SIMPLY VEGAN

THE COMPLETE STRESS-FREE GUIDE TO NAVIGATING A NEW VEGAN LIFESTYLE

VANESSA GARDENER

WWW.THEVEGANNOOK.COM

CONTENTS

To all animals
We hear you, we see you

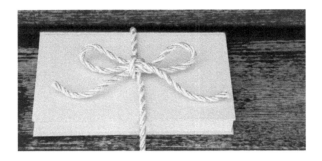

As a way to say thank you, we've put together The Essential Vegan Bundle, just for you.

Included are customizable recipes, the best resources and a grocer cheat sheet!

Click here for your bundle!

INTRODUCTION

So, you've heard about it on the news, on the latest Netflix documentary, or from your favorite Instagram influencer sharing their seemingly perfect life online between organic juice cleanses and farmers' market shopping hauls.

Veganism, the buzzword of the decade.

You might have dismissed it at first as if it was nothing but the hottest new trend booming among Millennials, health gurus, and hardcore dieters looking for a radical lifestyle change – one set to impress.

"Wait – can you really do that?"

"No meat, no eggs, no dairy... so, do they just eat salad all day?"

"What about cheese? I can't believe people would actually give up cheese!"

First, you are dumbfounded, then confused, and finally intrigued.

Several days of research later, and here you are, possibly for the first time, considering going vegan – maybe that's even the reason why you decided to pick up this book.

Does any of this sound familiar? Because that is my story and the story of thousands of other vegans spread around the globe.

When I first started looking into veganism, a whopping eight years ago, I was overwhelmed. I'm not only talking about the pages of contradicting information, such as the odd balance between the unfounded health claims of spiritual healers and the nutritional scaremongering of wary doctors.

I was overwhelmed by how many steps, tiny little transformations I would need to make to my routine in order to become vegan and do it right.

Going vegan encompasses so many aspects of our daily lives, more than those new to the lifestyle might realize. At least three times a day, avoiding meat, dairy, fish, and eggs is a choice we have to make. It's going to mean saying no to Friday night take-away with our non-vegan significant other (unless it's vegan, of course), saying no to a slice of birthday cake at your coworker's leaving party, or give away our favorite pair of leather boots to charity before we're ready to part from how comfortable they are.

Depending on the support system around you, going vegan might mean having to justify your lifestyle to a growing number of people every day. Although veganism has seen a surge in popularity in recent years, it's still far from being the norm. You might be feeling like you're supposed to have all the answers straight away and be ready to educate others at the drop of a hat. All the while, you are trying to manage your new vegan lifestyle, researching and experimenting all on your own.

Now that I think about it, overwhelming is quite the understatement!

Of course, I didn't have nearly the same amount of incredible vegan online resources available now, nor did I know any vegans in real life to approach for help and guidance. Even if I had all the resources and knowledge in the world, it wouldn't have made the transition any more easygoing.

The reason why going vegan can be such a monumental challenge for many of us comes down to one simple word: change.

Change is something all humans are afraid of, no matter how adventurous or daring they might be. It is embedded in our DNA, firmly planted in our subconscious, and at some point in our collective history, resistance to change was necessary to ensure our survival. We are hardwired to avoid risks and stick to a routine that keeps us content enough, even if we know it's not the best, even if we know a simple change could help us achieve so much more than what we are settling for now.

Veganism made complete sense to me: it was a practical change to my daily routine that meant I would no longer be directly contributing to the needless and senseless acts done to animals, a way in which I would positively affect the world and improve my life and health almost instantly in a way no other lifestyle could. As a nutritionist, I already had some background necessary to approach a vegan lifestyle healthily and consciously. Still, even when the reading was done and the sources triple-checked, more doubts would come to mind urging me to dive deeper.

Looking back, I regret not making a choice sooner. Still, the uncertainty and lack of a vegan community around me that could answer all the burning questions I had made it almost impossible to truly commit and say: *"Yes, I'm going vegan now."*

That's why I decided to write this book so that other lost new vegans and vegan-curious would have a handy guide to turn to when the change starts feeling too overwhelming, and the steps too confusing. Every reader can come to these first pages knowing nothing about veganism and reach the last page learning all the insights that seasoned, long-term vegans like me spent years discovering. I have gathered a collection of eye-opening scientific studies, filtered through my experience as a nutritionist, and personal accounts from vegans worldwide to create a chapter for every question you may have.

After years of helping friends and clients go vegan, one thing I've come to realize is that the more informed a choice is, the more people are comfortable to embrace the scary change and stick with their decisions in the long run, healthier and happier than ever.

In a way, I've found that knowledge and support are all you need to rewire your nature and look forward to the change you've been so afraid of.

We'll start things off by exploring the basics of vegan living, the history and principles of a vegan lifestyle, and what veganism looks like in 2020 and beyond.

We'll be diving into the tenets of optimal vegan nutrition for adults and children, the daily challenges vegans face in a non-vegan world, and what to expect when shopping, traveling or merely sharing your interest in the lifestyle with family, friends, and doctors!

Finally, here's a little disclaimer for those of you who are entirely new to the concept of veganism and are scared of what even the idea of a radical change might entail for your day-to-day life. I can't promise reading this book is all you're going to need to become vegan, but I can guarantee that it will give you all the tools you may need to start your vegan journey on the right foot.

If you've tried going vegan before but couldn't quite make it past the first few weeks or months: I recognize your struggle.

No matter how much you respect Joaquin Phoenix's unwavering vegan commitment, or how many times you've watched Leonardo DiCaprio's latest inspiring speech and documentary, going vegan is always going to present enough challenges to make giving up oh-so-tempting. I have been there before – but I also got past it.

I can promise that the information collected in this book will equip you with more than enough awareness to become the vegan example you strive to be. With a chapter for every challenge that might come your way, I can assure you that you'll be closing this book with a newfound passion and drive to become your best vegan self.

1

ALLOW ME TO INTRODUCE YOU

*I*t all started with milk.

I used to love milk. I was always eager to have a good glass of skim milk with my breakfast and a generous amount of froth in my morning coffee cup.

It's what makes your bones grow strong, after all – or at least, that's what my mother used to tell me every morning growing up, as she encouraged me to pour just a little more in my cereal.

However, in my early twenties, the taste of it started, inexplicably, to put me off. I wasn't aware of many things at that time, like the fact that almost 70% of the world's population is lactose intolerant.[1]

All I knew is that drinking milk stopped feeling like a treat; it was way too thick, overwhelmingly rich, and soon realized that my beloved lattes would often lead to some pretty bad bloating.

So, I decided to stop drinking dairy milk and picked up some soy milk instead. Much to my surprise, my digestive issues disappeared overnight.

This milk revelation was the catalyst to start diving deeper into the science of nutrition, leading me to study nutrition and think twice about my eating habits later on.

Soon after, I noticed that eating meat, be it chicken or beef, would also cause me to experience some less than ideal side effects. After every meat-heavy meal, I would become increasingly lethargic, often needing to take a short nap to recover and let the bloating go down.

If you've eaten meat all your life, you might think that the heavy, sluggish feeling you experience after a big meal is a normal, natural part of life.

Let me blow your mind: it's not! But I would only discover this after giving up meat and dairy entirely and becoming a vegetarian.

While eating eggs, legumes, and plenty of vegetables as my primary sources of calories made me feel a lot better, I knew I had to continue to look deeper, and eventually, I did. My mind had been opened to a different way of eating, and I was in full-on exploration mode, not ready to give up on my search anytime soon.

My next revelation came in the form of a Facebook post.

While scrolling through Facebook between activities one day, I came across a post from an old high school acquaintance, sharing the trailer for a new documentary: Forks Over Knives. The premise was enough to make me watch the full movie: can a healthy diet alone spare us some of the most dangerous diseases of our time? It turns out that the healthy diet promoted by the documentary was called veganism. While I had an idea of what the lifestyle was about from my research, I did not know what following a strict vegan diet would achieve.

From that moment on, I fell hard into the vegan rabbit hole.

I started to research all that I could about its origins, practices, and countless scientific studies detailing an animal product-free diet's benefits.

I soon realized it was way more than just a diet.

WHAT IS VEGANISM?

Veganism is a lifestyle that rejects the use of all animal products in every aspect of a person's life – well beyond diet alone.

For a long time, I thought being vegan was a modern concept, rooted in contemporary healthy eating practices and the current sustainability movement, but this philosophy goes back centuries.

Back then, vegans were called strict vegetarians instead, differing from vegetarians for their avoidance of animal-derived clothing, dairy products, and eggs in addition to meat and fish. For example, the Greek philosopher and mathematician Pythagoras advocated an early form of veganism as far back as 500 BC.[2]

Still, the words "vegan" and "vegetarian" were often synonymous with one another. In 1944, English vegan activist Donald Watson coined the term vegan to separate his lifestyle from the mainstream vegetarian movement.

The Vegan Society was founded in the same year, standing as one of the most influential and well-known vegan advocacy groups worldwide to this day. It is thanks to The Vegan Society that we have an official definition of what veganism is:

> *"A way of living which seeks to exclude, as far as is possible and practicable, all forms of exploitation of, and cruelty to, animals for food, clothing or any other purpose."*

There's quite a lot to unpack in this sentence alone.

Veganism defines the use of animals for food, clothing, or entertainment as exploitation – something most people rarely give much thought to.

I certainly never thought that using animals was cruel or exploitative. It is the standard; after all, it is merely the way things are, how our society has functioned for millennia.

The more I sat with that thought, however, the more uncomfortable I felt.

When animals' use is framed as exploiting other living beings, veganism's central belief starts to make sense.

No creature is more deserving of life than another.

Using animals and their by-products for food is deemed unnecessary, harmful, and cruel within this framework.

This framework brings us to the first question popping in most people's minds whenever they meet a vegan: *what on earth could you possibly eat?*

Vegans abstain from eating meat, fish, dairy, eggs, honey, and any other animal by-product. This abstinence takes out a massive chunk of a person's standard diet, which generally revolves around these products entirely.

Even though you might be thinking there is nothing left to eat, the world of vegan food is incredibly varied, colorful, and delicious. I'm willing to bet that you already consume a fair amount of vegan products daily: think rice, potatoes, beans, peanut butter, pasta, all types of fruit. These incredible foods are part of what vegans eat.

Don't worry — I will be expanding upon the joys of vegan food and what non- vegan products to watch out for in Chapter 4! For the time being, let this be a delicious spoiler of what's to come.

Another issue to tackle is animal exploitation in clothing, beauty, household items, and what exactly vegans strive to avoid when it comes to these products.

Leather, wool, suede, silk, down, and fur are also animal products. Meat and dairy by-products like gelatin and whey can be found in beauty and cosmetic products and seemingly animal-free groceries like candy and cereal bars. Products tested on animals also fall into the category of animal exploitation and cruelty – in the U.S., even sugar is not considered vegan-friendly![3]

Learning about veganism can open up your mind to the countless ways we use animals in our daily lives, beyond just eating meat, dairy, and eggs. It's a lifestyle choice that can impact all areas of a person's life, so it's only natural it would take a new vegan quite a lot of time to adjust to a 100% cruelty-free routine.

Let's have a little experiment to drive the point home.

Take a look at your living room: can you see a big leather couch or a couple of fluffy pillows?

Now, go inside your closet: are there any wool cardigans, leather bags, and wallets, or a pair of suede dress shoes you use for work? What about your deodorant, perfume, toothpaste, or favorite shampoo – do you know if their ingredients are free of animal products or that they weren't tested on animals?

These are just some examples of products vegans would not purchase or use, opting for vegan alternatives instead. Vegans will also avoid funding organizations or activities that exploit or harm animals in any way, such as circuses, aquariums, zoos, horse races, hunting, and fishing.

Now, this is where most people start feeling overwhelmed. I certainly did.

There are many steps, so many big and small changes, uprooting all that you knew by transforming lifelong habits... and for what? What makes so many of us take the leap and embrace veganism, with all of its struggles and challenges?

Even though there is no single right answer to this question, broadly speaking, there are three.

WHY VEGAN?

Before we continue, I wanted to mention that I didn't start calling myself a vegan right away.

Although veganism's core message deeply resonated with me and incorporating more and more plant-based meals into my diet became the norm, I wasn't sure I was wholly prepared to commit to this lifestyle.

Only when I understood the bigger picture, educating myself on why people choose to go vegan, that I felt ready to embark on my vegan journey proudly and openly.

Knowing your "why" is the key to understand what veganism is about, beyond definitions, semantics, and history lessons.

Vegan for the Animals

"Three times a day, I remind myself that I value life and do not want to cause pain to or kill other living beings. That is why I eat the way I do."

— NATALIE PORTMAN

There is a reason why I wanted to focus on the official definition of veganism - ethics are indeed the backbone of this lifestyle.

Not wanting to cause unnecessary harm to other beings is why veganism exists in the first place. A few decades down the line, the movement has grown to become more than an animal rights crusade, but its original message still brings many people worldwide to give up animal products from their diet and consumer choices.

Most people would classify themselves as animal lovers. All of you owning pets will know how much affection and joy your pup or kitten brings to your life and feel compelled to love and care for them in return.

From the moment we are born, we are taught to love some animals while eating others. We are taught that dogs, cats, and hamsters need our protection, while pigs, cows, and chickens do not deserve the same treatment.

Vegans reject this social norm. Those who do not follow the vegan lifestyle are often labeled as a product of collective *cognitive dissonance*. Complicated vocabulary aside, this means that there is a gap between their morals and actions: we love animals, yet we eat them.

We believe that killing is wrong, yet we end the lives of over 200 million land animals[4] every day. We appraise children for pulling at a lizard's tail yet choose to buy products made through the suffering of living, thinking creatures.

These are not simple realities to come to terms with, but it's not anyone's fault.

You most likely never had to hunt to feed yourself and your family or kill an animal you raised to have dinner for the day. It's easy to head down to your local grocery store and buy some chicken breast or a milk chocolate bar. In this modern, hyper-industrialized world, you have no choice but to be disconnected from the process it took for those products to get in your cart.

At this point, you might be asking yourself:

"Well, I can see why killing animals for meat and fish is cruel... but what about dairy and eggs? How are they cruel if animals don't die?"

It may be harder to see, but dairy and egg production are even crueler in many ways.

The reality is that dairy cattle are forcefully impregnated to produce milk and have their babies taken from them right after birth. The newborn calves are sent to the veal industry for slaughter, raised for more milk, or raised in harsh conditions for meat, and the process repeats for years on end. In the egg industry, male chicks are considered useless, so they are ground up alive, whereas females will be raised to spend their short lives cramped on top of one another in tiny cages, just like their mother hens.

Vegans have chosen to align their actions with their morals by refusing to support an industry that breeds, exploits, and kills animals for their commodities. In a vegan's eyes, a steak is a cow, breakfast bacon is a pig, and a carton of milk results from a baby calf being taken away from her mother.

Do you believe in doing your part to reduce the suffering of other creatures?

If the answer is yes, you might have taken your first step towards becoming an ethical vegan.

Vegan for the Environment

"We have a responsibility to act now to minimize our impact on this planet – for our children and future generations who will inherit what we leave behind."

— PAUL MCCARTNEY

One of the most compelling cases in support of veganism is the environmental argument.

The science is definite: going vegan is the single most effective way to reduce your carbon footprint,[5] making the world a far better place in the process.

In the last five years, we've seen a massive cultural shift towards sustainable living. From the collective rejection of single-use plastic to the decline of fast fashion, we collectively pull together to mitigate the climate crisis's consequences.

However, as great as this shift has been, the animal products industry remains the biggest threat to our environment.

In 2018, the United Nations named animal agriculture, specifically meat production, the world's most urgent problem.[6] Why?

Just think about these not-so-fun facts:

- It takes one-quarter of all of our freshwater to sustain the meat and dairy industry.[7]
- Animal agriculture is responsible for 14% of all greenhouse gas emissions.[8]
- Livestock feed has become the leading cause of deforestation, accounting for 91% of the Amazon rainforest's destruction.[9]

On the other hand, a person going vegan would save approximately 200,000 gallons of water a year,[10] cut CO_2 emissions by 70%,[11] and decrease land use by a whopping 76%, saving the rainforest and countless habitats in the process.[12]

And this is only the tip of the iceberg. Overfishing has led to permanent changes to the marine ecosystem, managing to reduce the total fish population by half compared to 1970[13] – that was only 50 years ago. The demand for "cheap fish" like tuna and mackerel, in particular, has become unsustainable, and the two species are currently on the brink of extinction in some places!

It isn't very comforting to think what another 50 years would do to our seas and oceans. After becoming aware of these numbers, I thought about the unnecessary damage my pre-vegan lifestyle inflicted upon the planet's ecosystem.

When pregnant with my second child, knowing all of this, the reality of climate change started to hit me for the first time – the earth is running out of time, and we created this catastrophe. How could I leave my kids with a better world if the world I knew would disappear by the time they were my age?

Learning about the significant impact that animal products have on climate change gave me the courage to call myself a vegan. I'm just a regular person: I can't pass laws, lobby for better environmental policies, or single-handedly put a stop to deforestation, water pollution, and world hunger.

But I can stand up for what I believe in by boycotting one type of the industries that pollute our planet the most, animal husbandry, and doing my part to guarantee my children have a future.

TRBUT26 | SIMPLY VEGAN

Vegan for Your Health

"Let food be thy medicine and medicine be thy food."

— HIPPOCRATES

Finally, we come to what many of you would consider a deal-breaker: veganism's health aspect. Whether cutting all animal products from your diet is actually good for you or a disaster that your body cannot recover from.

After all, the suffering of animals and the threats posed to our environment by animal agriculture could be argued if being vegan was unhealthy, dangerous, or in any way impracticable.

But as my personal experience and the experiences of countless other long-term vegans out there have shown, veganism is far from being unhealthy – according to science, it comes out on top as the optimal human diet.

Moreover, following a vegan diet is ideal for those suffering from heart disease, high blood pressure, diabetes, and obesity. Veganism has been shown to prevent these diseases from occurring, reduce and help manage their symptoms, and fully reverse them.[14] You might even know a couple of friends who decided to try cutting out animal products from their diet as a New

Year's resolution, seeing incredible benefits in weight management, energy, vitality, and overall health.

Are you looking to shed a pound or two? Vegans are consistently reported to have the lowest Body Mass Index.[15] Even when eating on a calorie surplus, vegans have been shown to maintain their weight much more efficiently than any other dieter following a calorie-restricted omnivorous diet.[16]

Are you looking to reduce your risk of cardiovascular issues? It's been shown that a vegan diet prevents and substantially reverses the life-threatening effects of America's number one killer – heart disease.[17]

A balanced, nutrient-dense vegan diet is safe for people of all ages, genders, and backgrounds. According to the Academy of Nutrition and Dietetics, vegan diets are healthful, nutritionally adequate, and beneficial for children as much as for adults – athletes included.[18] So whether you're a moderately active mother of two like me, a rising football star, or a growing teen, you can be sure you will thrive on a vegan diet if you take all the necessary precautions.

These include doing your research on what a balanced, health-promoting vegan diet looks like, eat enough calories to fuel your activity levels, and supplement essential vitamins and nutrients daily. Veganism can provide you with a blank slate to become the healthiest version of yourself you can be, and it's not uncommon to start seeing results in the first couple of weeks.

But what about protein, vitamin B_{12}, or any other essential nutrient commonly believed to be lacking in a vegan diet? Doesn't the need for supplementation undermine the argument that a plant-based diet is healthy and nutritionally adequate? Well, I'm going to be tackling those issues in Chapters 9 and 10, providing some much-needed myth-busting around these popular misconceptions.

I'll leave you with this: no vegan has ever been admitted to the hospital due to a protein deficiency, while thousands die every year in the U.S. alone due to animal product-related illnesses.

So you might as well give veganism a try, right?

2

BE COMPASSIONATE TO YOU

*I*t may feel like there are a lot of rules, routines, brand-new habits, nutritional guidelines, and moral talks.

Maybe you've had a few friends reacting to your interest in veganism with skepticism, telling you how hard it's going to be. You might have experienced some criticism or teasing from your family, who don't seem to share the same passion for nutrition, sustainability, or ethics.

I was met with a similar kind of resistance when I first shared interest in the vegan lifestyle with my parents and older brother. They had never researched the topic and were "stuck in their ways" when it came to tradition and habits. A close childhood friend of mine, who oddly enough started looking into a plant-based lifestyle around the same time that I did, shared the same experience:

> *"I was confused and hurt, and couldn't understand why the people that were so close to me could not understand where I was coming from. I never asked them to come on this journey with me, but in a way, maybe that's how I came across when I was arguing so passionately about why going vegan was so important to me and the world at large. Still, the lack of support got to me at first. Since I didn't know any other vegans in my small town, I started to feel increasingly overwhelmed by all the conflicting information I was getting. Veganism looked like a goal I couldn't achieve, so I just kept researching and researching without taking any actions for months".*

Not having the support you need when going through something so life-changing as adopting a vegan lifestyle can make or break a new vegan. In this case, it almost broke us, preventing us from starting our vegan journey much later than we probably would have if there'd have been a friendly, trustworthy guide holding our hand through it.

If going vegan is already beginning to sound like the most difficult challenge you've ever considered tackling in your life, it's tempting to give up before even starting. The number of people who return to eating animal products after a short (or even longer) period of being vegan is overwhelmingly large,[1] after all.

So how can we take action to prevent becoming part of this number too?

The key is compassion. Although we have gone over the topic of kindness to animals quite extensively when discussing veganism, we have yet to touch on a more fundamental type of empathy: the one you owe to yourself.

Forget about the snarky comments and skepticism from family and peers, forget about the anti-vegan articles you might have seen around on the web, and forget about the little voice inside your head that might be telling you you're not strong enough to succeed.

Now is your chance to begin a purpose-led life with a fresh slate and completely revolutionize how you experience the world around you. Even though the world has become a more vegan-friendly place than ten years ago, many of you won't have a vegan best friend or a reliable support system around you to make the transition easier. Having no support could be a once in a lifetime opportunity to discover how strong and self-reliant you can be, using only the power of your motivation and beliefs to become who you aspire to be.

I want to share five tips that have helped me get into a more positive mindset as I took my first steps towards veganism, which ultimately allowed me to approach this transition in a relaxed, stress-free, and even fun way.

KEEP AN OPEN MIND

What exactly is the meaning of open-mindedness?

Being open-minded means being open, with no exception, to all possibilities and experiences. It means refusing to take things at face value, questioning all the things you take for granted, and being receptive to learning new things by getting out of your comfort zone. In the context of becoming vegan, it means being open to change. It means not being scared of creating new habits, dropping lifelong routines, taking in brand-new information free of bias.

If you're entirely new to veganism, many of the facts and philosophical views expressed in the last chapter left you scratching your head, though quite possibly not.

If going vegan is so beneficial to the environment, why are governments not acting to discourage meat consumption? If going vegan can reverse so many life-threatening conditions, why has my doctor never mentioned it before? Hint: It's money!

These are reasonable questions to ask at this point; so many truths about the way we produce and consume animal products seem unbelievable. But couldn't it be possible that our politicians and doctors would also fail to keep an open mind and refuse to accept differing opinions and bombshell facts that challenge their unshakable worldview? Even with all the possible changes, these truths would entail?

While many think of open-mindedness as a character trait, it is more of a skill that anybody can learn, luckily. Mastering this skill is essential to starting your unique vegan journey, whether you're considering the lifestyle for dietary or ethical reasons.

The key is implementing accommodation into your thought process. In psychological terms, accommodation is the process that occurs in our minds as we learn new information challenging what we already know.[2] This can be difficult, but it can become much more natural with repetition – and with three main techniques to help you.

1. Share What You Have Learned With a Neutral Party

There's never any shame in asking for help under any circumstances. As you start to intake new information challenging firmly held beliefs about nature and society, like that we need animal products to live, make sure you turn to a neutral party to get an objective view of the two opposing points.

A neutral party can be a therapist, a school counselor, or even an inanimate object like a journal if you feel like there's nobody you can personally approach. Sharing allows you to divulge the new challenging information you've learned and your conflicting thoughts to a non-judgmental person. They can help give you an objective look at the situation.

The accommodation process can lead to either confusion or denial, and more frequently, a decent mix of the two. Having your thoughts laid out in front of you can help clarify what you've learned and your position on the matter, allowing you to tap into your logic and intuition without any external influence.

Try this exercise with one of the "why vegan" points I have explored in the last chapter, maybe the one your mind feels most uncomfortable with. Research it in full, double-check all sources, and finally explain it aloud to a neutral party, or scribble in a journal or a smartphone's notes app. This is the first step toward providing clarity and uncovers any subconscious or conscious biases you may have, stemming from your personality, socialization, or life experience.

2. Reframe Your Thoughts and Fight the Confirmation Bias

The next step in making accommodation easier is reframing negative views and opinions you've laid out and become aware of your biases.

Becoming aware takes a lot of intellectual humility. Confirmation bias, the cognitive process that subconsciously takes place in your brain as you learn new information, leads you to choose a "right" and "wrong" according to what you already believe is right or wrong from previous experience or knowledge.[3]

In simpler terms, this process leads you to agree to facts that are already supported by your deeply held beliefs and discount the information that goes against them – even if the conflicting information is objectively more credible. This process is fundamentally the root of all close-mindedness.

I'll give you an example from my vegan journey. As I started exploring the ethical side of veganism, I found out that cows milk was unnatural for humans to consume. It was also the product of artificial insemination, forced pregnancy, and veal slaughter was incredibly troubling to me. What I was seeing was something I could hardly believe despite being shown undercover footage of milk production and despite listening to countless personal accounts of ex farmworkers.

So my mind tried to rectify this discomfort by denying it all.

"Maybe this happens in other countries, but it would never happen here!"

"Cows need to be milked; otherwise, they'll suffer!"

"There must be a reason why we need milk... there's no way this industry could've gone for this long if there wasn't any need for it!"

I had already given up on milk and cheese after experiencing digestive issues. However, I still believed that cow milk was healthy for most people but also the product of a very natural process. I had been under the assumption that cows produce milk around the clock and need humans to milk them – so using that milk for food wasn't wrong.

No one ever challenged that assumption. The truth about dairy milk wasn't explained to me in school as I learned about biology or visited my first small farm on a school trip.

Cows, like any other mammal, have to be pregnant to produce milk. That milk is meant for their child to grow, and no one else – especially not for an entirely different species!

It was logical, it was realistic, and it made perfect sense. Still, I couldn't let myself believe it without coming up with argument after argument. Only when I shared my confusion and disbelief with my journal could I look at the information more objectively. After asking more questions and looking into more research, I finally concluded that what I previously thought was accurate was instead a big lie, fed to me by a mix of propaganda and ignorance.

With time, I even started to notice little pieces of this propaganda divulged by the media: the image of the happy farm and the laughing cow, the "got milk?" posters, the "essential" portions of milk on the "milk order form" that was brought home by my son from school.

I had to slowly let go of the doubt and disbelief, fight confirmation bias, recognize my cognitive dissonance, and reframe my view entirely. Then I applied this method to everything else I felt uncomfortable about – and here I am.

Now, this is easier said than done. Cognitive dissonance, or more generally, accommodating ideas that challenge your existing beliefs, is challenging. The process might take some time to become comfortable enough to confront your bias. Or you may even be thinking, *"how could I have been blind for so long?"*. That's okay too.

Many people never get the opportunity to challenge their beliefs head-on, and the ones who do get the chance, like you and me, live to become better people because of it. At the end of the day, you don't necessarily have to change your view on anything – even just attempting to open your mind to different possibilities will make you grow.

3. Get Out of Your Comfort Zone

Getting outside of the comfort zone is a great exercise that will improve all areas of your life, and it can also be an invaluable tool for practicing open-mindedness.

Think about a time when you said "yes" to something you never tried before. Despite some initial anxiety, you'll likely find the new experience to be quite fun, transformative, and, most importantly, mind-opening!

Getting out of your comfort zone will impact how you see the world – even if you're not aware of it. Whether it's going to a concert that is far out of your music taste, meeting new people from different backgrounds, traveling, or merely trying a brand-new dish from an exotic restaurant down the street.

Experiencing new things is what helps us grow by teaching us to embrace discomfort. As "taking risks" often turns out to be rewarding (such as making new friends or discovering a passion for a different music genre), we train our brain to open up to new possibilities much more quickly and easily.

The next time you're invited to a party where you're unlikely to know anybody, you'll find yourself saying yes with much less hesitation. At least once a week, try getting out of your comfort zone in a small way – no need to look up bungee jumping just yet. This change will already go a long way in reshaping your brain and slowly turning accommodation into a habit.

The way you see veganism will likely be impacted by this exercise as well. Embarking on a one-month vegan challenge, for example, will sound much more achievable and exciting when you are already used to trying new things every week. As habit is what ultimately informs most human behavior,[4] it won't be long until your one-month challenge turns into a lifelong lifestyle, if done consciously and most importantly, slowly.

TAKE IT SLOW

I believe I've made it quite clear that I took my sweet time before adopting a vegan lifestyle and before identifying as a vegan in front of others. Although I somewhat regret not making that choice sooner, the logical side of me knows I did the right thing – and some exciting data is backing me up on this too!

Whichever the reason you have decided to go vegan, I understand you might be looking forward to going all in and jumping into this lifestyle change as soon as possible, especially after overcoming closed-mindedness.

However, the key to staying vegan long-term is to make the transition as seamless and as attainable as possible. You don't have to be a zero-waste, smoothie-obsessed health guru or an all-around expert on veganism to join the movement in a significant way. Just start small and gradually build up on that!

According to a 2017 study, a staggering 84% of vegans and vegetarians end up going back to meat,[5] citing an inadequate diet, and social ostracizing as the main reasons. These are very humbling statistics, but you can avoid becoming part of this data by taking it easy and slow – "overnight" vegans often lack the necessary preparation to stick to the long-term lifestyle.

What makes me say that? Well, last night, I opened my inbox asking fellow vegans to share their transition timeline, and I noticed a pattern:

"I went vegan right away, and yet it took me about a year to completely stop eating animal products, especially when going to restaurants with my non-vegan friends."

"I went vegan overnight and wish I would've waited longer... transitioning from an Omni diet to a full vegan one isn't easy – it felt like a shock to the body."

Of course, not all the replies I received involved flip-flopping or hardship, but the volume was enough to conclude that a gradual progression towards veganism can be more sustainable — slow and steady wins the race.

Tackle the most apparent challenge first, your diet, and break it down into more manageable steps. An example would be to cut out all red meat from your diet first, let a week or two pass, and then move onto cutting out chicken, then fish, dairy, and eggs. Remember that this is *your* timeline. It is *your* time to reflect on your choices and build new habits that'll last for a lifetime – how fast or how slow you will progress will only depend on how you feel, free from any external pressure.

Time management is going to be crucial. Allocate some time, every week, to learn new recipes, discover new restaurants, and journal about your experience. Planning your meals and shopping trips will also be extremely beneficial – the display of chocolate bars waiting for you at checkout might become too tempting if you let yourself get distracted or hungry!

Once you feel confident in your full plant-based diet plan, you might want to incorporate other veganism aspects that resonate with you. Try getting rid of old clothes and accessories made from animals, like leather shoes and woolen scarves, by either donating them to charity or gifting them to a friend. Start buying certified cruelty-free and vegan makeup and toiletries and replace them right away, or substitute them as they run out.

Making one small change a week will ensure you are consistently pushing yourself out of your comfort zone, but not so much you feel overwhelmed and stressed out by the constant change in routine.

BE PREPARED — BUT GIVE YOURSELF A BREAK

While you commit to adopting a vegan diet, make sure you are fully ready to tackle your nutritional needs and cravings head-on.

The first thing I suggest doing is going online and researching all the big grocery stores and vegan eateries near you. You might be surprised by how many vegan-friendly options are in your area or disappointed by the inadequate amount. In that case, you may wish to do some extra planning to make sure you have everything you need for your first month of plant-based eating – but don't worry, you'll be able to find vegan staples in every big supermarket.

Your first shopping trip will likely involve stocking up on those staples (plus plenty of plant-based snacks for those pesky midnight cravings). We are talking about rice, potatoes, oats, pasta, cans of beans, lentils, nuts, seeds, plenty of spices, frozen and fresh vegetables and fruits.

I will be discussing vegan food and vegan nutrition extensively in later chapters. Still, in the meantime, I recommend you download vegan food blogger *Pick Up Limes'* free pdf grocery guide[6] for a first look at how your weekly shopping will look (check out their website). You'll soon discover that a healthy, budget-friendly vegan diet is much more accessible than you might have thought, so there's no need to travel miles to shop at a Whole Foods branch!

However, in terms of extensive research and conscious grocery shopping, preparation can only go so far. Likely, you will accidentally eat some animal products on a night out with relatives. It's okay to mess up and make mistakes – you're still human, and you're still learning.

You might misread the ingredients label for a new snack bar you picked up last minute or eat something non-vegan by mistake as your dietary requirements get lost in translation when traveling. It's all part of the vegan process, and we need to make mistakes to learn from them, so we can hopefully educate ourselves and others in the long run.

Give yourself a break! It might take longer than you initially expected to switch to a vegan diet entirely, but as long as you're doing your best and doing all that you can to be knowledgeable and prepared, you're doing it right. Being too hard on yourself over some unexpected gelatin won't make the world a better place, but staying strong in your beliefs and powering through genuine mistakes will.

TAP INTO YOUR WHY POWER

What happens if you're still finding yourself unable to commit to your decision after all the pep talk, research, and shopping trips?

What happens when you struggle to follow through with what you believe?

In my experience, these things happen when we find ourselves disconnected from our core values. If you have just recently decided to adopt veganism as a core value, it will take some time for your actions to align with your mind seamlessly as any other belief you've nurtured your whole life. It will more than likely require some effort on your part to remind yourself of what being vegan means to you.

This process is called setting your why power:[7] actively reminding yourself of your core values and why they are essential. What is the reason you've decided to give veganism a try, and how does that reason connect your core values? These are questions you need to be able to answer before moving forward.

Your reason for starting on the vegan path can vary and still end up exactly where all other vegans are — holding the belief that no animal should suffer and actively practicing to align with that. I went plant-based initially for health but came around to veganism later. Right now, your reasons may be for more vitality, a healthier body, or even climate change, though remember that veganism at its core is about the animals. No matter where we start, it's still a benefit to them and ourselves, which is a win all around.

One of the best ways to naturally reinforce your why power is to have constant reminders around you. These reminders can take the form of post-it notes posted around the house (with particular attention to the kitchen area), journal or online blog entries, or even simple pop-up reminders on your phone. You can try leaving short, supportive messages to yourself, encouraging you to face the challenges on your path with confidence, or even better, filling your living space with inspiring facts and quotes about veganism and plant-based nutrition.

I encourage you to continue this exercise even after your transition to a vegan lifestyle comes to an end. Every once in a while, my long-term vegan friends and I still have little get-togethers to watch our favorite vegan documentaries, so we can remind ourselves of why we do the things we do and why our lifestyle matters to us. As time goes on, it's incredibly easy to become disconnected from your core values and somewhat forget where your why power lies.

BE UNAPOLOGETICALLY YOU

"Nothing has changed my life more. I feel better about myself as a person, being conscious and responsible for my actions. I lost weight, my skin cleared up, I got bright eyes, and I just became stronger, healthier, and happier. I can't think of anything better in the world to be but be vegan."

— ALICIA SILVERSTONE

At last, here is my final piece of advice: never forget to be unapologetically *you*.

No vegan journey will look the same for two people. The time it takes you to transition fully will depend on your personality, adaptation skill, and different external factors like community support. Every way that will lead you to veganism is valid, and any amount of time it'll take you to adopt the lifestyle into your diet or purchase choices is right – just right for you.

I encourage you to try these tips for yourself and the more practical tools for success that I'm going to present in the next chapter, in any way that works for you. You might even decide that the slow, gradual progression towards veganism is not the right fit for you, preferring to go vegan overnight. You might not struggle with the accommodation process as much, or you might find that it will take much more time and conscious learning to get out of your comfort zone.

You're welcome to create your path and blueprint for how you will go vegan; that's the whole point. Don't let anybody tell you you're doing things wrong when you're just following your flow and believe that countless other vegans out there, and I will support you in whatever direction you choose.

3

SETTING UP FOR SUCCESS

*Y*ou are now well-equipped with valuable psychological tools to get started on a vegan life-style in the most stress-free way. It's now time to look into how to implement those tools and transform them into practical, effective action.

Here I'll explain how you can set yourself up for success.

I will explore the types of routines you can set up from the get-go, how to create the perfect home environment for change, and how to surround yourself with the right support system and media environment to succeed as a new vegan without all the hassle you're probably dreading.

These tips are taken from a mix of my personal experience and the experiences of other inspiring vegans I have met along the way. If you're an ex-smoker or have kicked another habit, you might already be familiar with some self-help techniques. These are designed to aid you in crucial moments of transition, moments where your surroundings and daily rituals can either make or break a new positive habit.

THE MAGIC OF ROUTINES AND RITUALS

In his 2012 smash-hit *The Power of Habit*, business reporter Charles Duhigg identifies how daily, often every day habits can affect our behavior (and, in turn, our whole lives) by effectively changing patterns inside our brains.[1]

According to the scientific findings informing this book, the key to achieving all of our goals, be it exercising regularly, becoming more productive, achieving success in our careers, or changing our diet, is understanding how habits work. Tweaking and changing our habits can make even the most demanding challenges effortless.

In short, habits are not just what we do – they define who we are.

That's why setting a routine and ritual to follow every day or a few times weekly is crucial to establishing long-term mindsets and lifestyles. Think of this step as a way of reprogramming your brain: just like children learn to follow basic routines to grow and develop, you will be embarking on a similar journey as an adult by introducing new, simple habits designed to get you closer to your goal – in this case, happy and healthy life as a vegan.

Let's start from the very beginning with setting up a morning routine. Whether you're aware of it or not, you already have an established ritual you follow diligently every morning, like brushing your teeth as soon as you're up, checking your phone for the latest news, or making a cup of coffee to start your day on the right foot.

So, what kind of morning rituals can we introduce into our routine to help us become the vegans we want to be?

I have found that morning journaling, writing down your reflections and intentions for the day ahead, can be extremely beneficial when transitioning to a vegan diet. I used to wake up craving fresh coffee every day and made the conscious choice to pair the existing ritual with this brand new one. As I sat in front of my kitchen table, sipping my almond milk latte and reflecting on my to-do list, I would write down a list of bullet points, setting my intentions for the day:

"I will nourish my body with whole, vegan foods today to feel healthy, energized, and motivated to study."

"I will organize a get-together with my friends and cook a delicious plant-based dinner for everybody, so I can show them how delicious a vegan diet can be"

If you're not keen on picking up a pen first thing in the morning, positive affirmations can play a very similar role. Try practicing daily affirmations in front of a mirror while brushing your teeth or getting dressed as doing so will help to incorporate them seamlessly into your existing routine:

> *"I believe Veganism is the best way of making a positive contribution to the planet, and I'll lead by example by making my vegan diet as sustainable as it can be"*

> *"I follow a healthful vegan diet because I believe in preventing life-threatening diseases so that I can be healthy for the sake of my children and loved ones."*

Chances are you're going to feel a bit silly while doing this – but don't worry, it's going to feel much more intuitive and natural as time goes on!

Light exercise or meditation has also been shown to promote a long-lasting sense of discipline and motivation. These can help keep you on track throughout the day. Instead of waking up and lying in bed while checking your phone for half an hour (I know, we're all guilty of this), try practicing breath-controlled light stretching or a five-minute meditation session. The key to making this exercise work is to clear your mind of all doubts and worries and focus on your breathing — no need to overthink this! This practice will allow you to feel refreshed and lighter, subconsciously directing you towards healthier, more mindful choices throughout the day.

Evening routines are just as important. Dinnertime is usually the best time to dedicate to cooking or meal prepping, as we are generally less busy or in less of a rush to move onto our next task. While occupied cooking your plant-based meal, you can let your mind wander and reflect on how the day went, on your little successes or mistakes, and set your intentions for the following day.

Remember to focus more on the positive aspects of your day rather than what you perceive to be failures or mistakes – positive reinforcement can truly work wonders, and beating yourself up over a slip-up won't do you any favors.

Finally, we have weekly routines, encompassing everything from Sunday afternoon meal prepping to grocery shopping. I encourage you to devote one day each week to plan and prepare plant-based meals in bulk. Suppose hours in the kitchen sounds incredibly daunting already. In that case, I completely understand where you're coming from. I'm far from being the best cook or the most passionate connoisseur. Oddly enough, preparing my meals in advance has made things much easier for me, saving me quite a bit of money (and sanity) at the end of each month.

Prepping a few days ahead of time is not only a great way to take inventory for grocery shopping (which you're going to need during the first few months as a vegan), but it can also help you track your daily nutrition intake. By getting all your food sorted in one go, you'll be avoiding one of the worst scenarios for a new vegan: coming home exhausted after a long day to an empty fridge or a pantry full of raw ingredients that might take hours to put together and cook.

Trust me – as a new vegan, you don't want to be in that position.

Meal planning and food prepping will allow you to create healthy plant-based meals that will get you the nutrients you need, get used to a new way of cooking, know what to shop for, and save a substantial amount of money all at once. Try making this routine as fun and easy as possible: invite family members or friends to cook with you, play some music, or let a movie play in the background. You will have days worth of meals before realizing it and grow to like spending time in the kitchen.

Last but not least, don't give up on practicing self-compassion.

There is no scientifically proven timeline when it comes to developing new habits. The idea that it takes us 21 days to form a new habit is fundamentally a myth,[2] despite being a prevalent cliché. Be kind to yourself by knowing that every little action you're taking today makes tomorrow easier, and encourage yourself to power on by looking at how far you've come from who you were yesterday.

CLEANSE, DECLUTTER, AND REMOVE ALL TEMPTATIONS

The next step in setting yourself up for success is creating an external environment that will encourage you and help you follow your new vegan diet. Naturally, the first place you might want to start with is the kitchen.

Having easy and complete access to various things from a previous lifestyle can be a surefire way to fall back into our old habits. When your cupboard and fridge still contain milk chocolate, cheese, chicken ramen, or any other non-vegan snack, it's much easier to say to yourself, *"come on, it's just this once,"* instead of sticking to your vegan principles. Your diet will be so much easier to follow if you decide to remove those temptations entirely while helping build a sense of trust within yourself that will prove you really can do this (and I know you can).

Start by clearing out your kitchen cupboards, pantry, fridge, and freezer of all non-vegan items. Doing this means getting rid of all meat and fish products, dairy products like cow milk and cheese, eggs, and honey, and double-checking the ingredients of all snacks and processed food you might have around for sneaky animal by-products. If you're not exactly sure what you should be watching out for, you can have a quick look at Chapter 6 for a comprehensive list.

Once you have successfully eliminated all animal products from your kitchen (or from the secret snack stash in your bedroom), you can decide whether you want to clear out other animal products from your environment. A quick tip: if a food item has cholesterol in the nutrition facts list, it contains an animal ingredient. If you feel that it's time to fully commit to a vegan lifestyle or take your first steps towards it, you can make a powerful statement of intention by cleaning out your closet and bathroom of non-vegan items. This means getting rid of all leather clothes, shoes, accessories, and wool, silk, suede, down, and fur items. You will then look at your toiletries or beauty products, researching their company's policy regarding animal testing. Carefully review the ingredients of each product you purchase (Chapter 6 will have a list).

This step might be quite hard for some, not just because you will actively get rid of products you have probably enjoyed for a long time.

Nobody likes being wasteful. The idea of tossing perfectly "good" food, giving away clothes in perfect condition, or getting rid of new body spray will likely sound pointless to you or even downright wrong.

When it comes to this issue, and others for that matter, not all vegans think the same. Some might choose to wear out their non-vegan clothes or consume all non-vegan toiletries and makeup to reduce waste. Others will see donating animal products or giving non-vegan food away as enforcing the idea that using animals for food or products is okay when they genuinely believe it is not.

Only you can decide where you stand on this. I can only reassure you that physically throwing away animal products will push your brain to think of them as repulsive. They will be so unnecessary that you not only wouldn't want to use them yourself but also wouldn't want anyone else to consume. It's a powerful statement, a meaningful way of setting your *why power* and sharing it with the world. The question of what's to be done with your old non-vegan products is still an ongoing debate within the vegan movement, but ultimately, it is your conscience that will decide for you.

BUILD A SUPPORT SYSTEM AND POSITIVE SOCIAL MEDIA

We live in a very non-vegan world. Although the movement has undoubtedly come leaps and bounds from its humble fringe beginnings, being a vegan is still far from being the norm, so you have to be aware that the world at large will not cater to your needs or think about your lifestyle the way you do. If it did, well, then everybody would be vegan already. Wouldn't that be amazing?

Your lifestyle is more than what you eat or what you choose to buy – it is also who you choose to have around. The final step in setting up for success is to create a supportive, vegan-friendly environment that will make you feel welcomed and understood.

Take a long, hard look at your inner circle (friends, family, partner, coworkers), reflect on how they support you through your vegan journey, and recognize if any of their behavior is influencing you negatively. If you find out that, upon reflection, some people in your life have you feeling uncomfortable or somewhat judged for your decision to go vegan, you might decide to limit the time you spend around them.

Of course, I am not saying you should cut all contacts with every important person in your life who's not vegan – for most of us, that would mean cutting connections with pretty much everyone we know. The majority of these people will be supportive of your lifestyle as it is making you happy and pushing you to become a better person, even if they don't necessarily connect with the vegan message the same way you do. You're not entering a cult. You are just making the conscious choice to live according to your true beliefs. Anyone who truly loves you is going to be supportive of that.

Still, the harsh reality is that there might be a small minority of acquaintances (or even close friends and family members) who will make your vegan transition much harder than necessary. Every vegan I know has faced some degree of mockery, judgment, or adverse comments directed towards their vegan lifestyle and a plant-based diet.

Just ask yourself this: why should you dedicate valuable time to people that make you feel awful for a choice that's not hurting anyone?

Transitioning to a vegan lifestyle can be hard enough for many of us. The quality of the support system we have around us through this time is going to be crucial. Support and understanding will lift and encourage us to keep going. Simultaneously, a cynical, hostile social environment can potentially break us and have us question our intentions or be ashamed of our beliefs.

Speaking from personal experience, you will do well by getting rid of toxic people in all aspects of your life, not just when veganism is involved. I understand if distancing yourself from unhealthy close contacts sounds incredibly scary, as we are always taught to be polite, understanding, and patient at all times — no matter how rude or hostile others are to us. If you're looking for greater insight on toxicity in our social environment, I suggest you pick up Al Bernstein's, *Emotional Vampires* for a very eye-opening read.

Now, our external environment doesn't end with just our social contacts. It is also reflected in the places we visit, the activities we take part in, and the media we consume. While transitioning to a vegan lifestyle, you might find that some of your favorite activities won't be as enjoyable as you remembered. Your trip to SeaWorld, a visit to your local pizza restaurant with friends, Friday night drinks and snacks with your coworkers might all start to sound less and less appealing the more you commit yourself to your new lifestyle. Fortunately for us, being vegan doesn't mean being a total social recluse.

It might be time to start researching vegan events in your area. Try connecting with your local plant-based community online or in real life, maybe as part of an activism effort, a round of educational talks, or just a visit to the new vegan restaurant. Social media is the first place you should head to if you're looking for fellow vegans or vegan events close to you, but websites like *Meetup.com* might also be worth a shot. There may even be a VegFest event coming up within the year (depending on where you live). VegFest is a worldwide vegan festival and plant-based food fair that is guaranteed to make you feel welcomed and seen, especially as a new vegan. Try heading over to *VegEvents.com* for a quick look at what events might be coming up.

Last but not least, start paying closer attention to the media you consume as well. In the golden age of social media, we are constantly bombarded by information, advertisement, and media content that can subtly influence how we see the world with a simple click. While keeping an open mind is always crucial to grow and improve ourselves, there is such a thing as surrounding yourself with potentially harmful and malicious information.

Harmful sources could include a YouTube channel you have subscribed to that keeps putting out meat-heavy recipes, a yogurt commercial you can't skip, or a show promoting an omnivorous diet as the only healthy diet. Whatever the source, lacking a balance of vegan-friendly media and information is the perfect recipe for vegan isolation.

We cannot avoid all non-vegan content, but it is paramount that you feel part of a vegan-friendly conversation as you take your first steps into a plant-based lifestyle. Following vegan-friendly media will educate you further and keep you in the veg loop and make you feel accepted and validated in your beliefs, especially if you don't yet have any vegan friends to reach out to.

Start following vegan Instagram accounts, subscribe to YouTube channels for recipe inspiration, subscribe to vegan newsletters for vegan news updates, and engage with this content as much as possible. Doing so will have you feel like part of a real community, no matter how far or how early you might be in your transition.

I recommend checking out accounts like *PlantBasedNews*, *TotalVeganBuzz*, and *VeganCommunity* on Instagram for vegan-related news, light-hearted memes, and lifestyle tips, and online publications like *Viva! Life*, *Veg News Magazine*, *Vegan Life Magazine*, and *Vegan Food & Living*. When it comes to YouTube, choices are abundant, with countless bloggers and content creators documenting their lives as vegans and sharing delicious recipes and valuable lifestyle tips. The channels I would most recommend for new vegans are *Hot For Food*, *Pick Up Limes*, *Cheap Lazy Vegan*, *Simnett Nutrition*, and *Mic The Vegan*.

In a non-vegan world, there will always be something that can anger or upset us, things we have little to no control over. However, making your environment more vegan-friendly is a foolproof way of feeling supported and validated in your decision. You're set for success before you even start cooking your first entirely plant-based meal.

And speaking of meals, I think it's finally time to address the awkward elephant in the room: what on earth are you going to eat as a vegan?

4

FOOD — THE GOOD STUFF

*L*et's get to the good stuff: food. Even as I gave up dairy milk and meat in a heartbeat and found my health much better for it, I struggled to imagine what my diet would look like without any animal products.

And trust me, I was so wrong in thinking that my life as a vegan would be flavorless and monastic – I never knew just how delicious food could be until I went vegan.

WHAT NOT TO EAT

Before we dive into the varied, colorful world of plant-based food, let's reiterate what makes some food items vegan and what types of food and ingredients vegans avoid so as not to betray their beliefs. Consider this a brief guide about what *not* to eat, but keep in mind that sneaky animal ingredients can be found in even the most plant-based-looking snack, and subtle animal products are also used in makeup, toiletries, and cleaning products. I'll be going over all the more subtle non-vegan ingredients in Chapter 6.

Now, I bet you may be thinking that going vegan will mean losing out on an endless list of products. Still, if you stop and reflect on the variety of foods available, you will soon realize that animal products make up a tiny percentage of food products.

Meat and poultry — This includes all types of meat like beef, pork, lamb, veal, horse, rabbit, wild game, and all kinds of poultry like chicken, turkey, and duck. Keep in mind that some meat products are sometimes hidden. For example, seemingly vegan-friendly vegetable ramen noodles might contain chicken stock.

Fish — This includes all types of fish (such as salmon, tuna, mackerel, or cod) and shellfish and crustaceans like shrimp and crab. Fish products can also be hidden in seemingly vegan-friendly products: traditional Worcester sauce, for example, contains anchovies.

Dairy products — Milk, cheese, yogurt, butter, cream, and several dairy by-products like whey and casein are often included in popular snack foods. Dairy products are relatively standard in almost all traditional baked goods, dressings, ice cream, or even bread.

Eggs — This doesn't only include whole eggs but also egg whites, often found as a binding agent in snack foods. Much like dairy, eggs can be found in almost all baked goods, salad dressings, and many noodle and pasta brands.

Honey and bee products — Bee-derived products generally tend to be overlooked when considering what vegans won't eat, but they're as much an animal product as milk or eggs. Besides honey, vegans will avoid royal jelly, bee pollen, and beeswax, commonly used in different medications.

WHAT TO EAT

Don't worry. You're in for a treat.

I have noticed that most people going vegan for the first time will often focus on what they're losing or missing out on rather than what they are gaining with their vegan transition. I know first-hand that "restriction" can be a scary word when adopting a plant-based diet. That's why I recommend adding to your diet first before taking anything away from it, or at least, make sure you have a plant-based substitute ready for every food item you're going to stop eating next.

I'm not exaggerating when saying there are plenty of delicious alternatives around, many of which you might have never heard of, so you know this will be an exciting ride. Being aware of this abundance is what I mean by "gaining something" – you will open your mind to many new foods, recipes, and flavor combinations that'll make your old diet staples pale in comparison.

The following are some examples of what you can eat as a vegan:

Legumes — These are varied, delicious, and incredibly healthy for you. You can always rely on legumes like kidney beans, lentils, chickpeas, black beans, soybeans (including tofu and tempeh), butter beans, peanuts, peas, split peas, and many more to keep you full and satisfied as a vegan.

Grains — Grains are a staple for many of us, and you'll find yourself basing your meals around these products even more as a vegan. This category includes wheat products like pasta, noodles, bread, rice, oats, corn, barley, rye, quinoa, millet, and many more.

Vegetables — If you were thinking nothing but romaine lettuce, think again. There are so many vegetables available globally (over a thousand) it'd be impossible to scratch the surface here, but I will do my best to name some common ones. Here are some: potatoes, sweet potatoes, pumpkin, zucchini, eggplant, tomatoes, spinach, collard greens, kale, beetroot, butternut squash, sweetcorn, peppers, carrots, snap peas, broccoli, cauliflower, celery, cucumbers, fennel, onions, garlic, and okra. You're guaranteed to find something you'll love within this list.

Fruits — The fruit list is just as big as the vegetable list, spanning from avocado and olives to strawberries, apples, bananas, melons, oranges, and peaches. Dried fruit is also a staple for many, with raisins, dates, cranberries, dried apricots, and figs, to name a few.

Nuts, seeds, and nut butter — Nuts and seeds are a nutritional powerhouse for vegans and are incredibly versatile. They are great if consumed on their own or added to exciting recipes such as vegan sauces, desserts, and cheeses (cashew cheese, for example). Nuts you might enjoy including walnuts, pecans, almonds, cashews, and pistachios. While peanuts and peanut butter are technically considered legumes, it'd be crazy not to have them on this list as well. Sunflower seeds, pumpkin seeds, hemp seeds, chia seeds, sesame seeds, and flax seeds are just some examples of delicious and heart-healthy ingredients vegans incorporate in their daily meals.

Mock meats and dairy vegan alternatives — As veganism steps further into the mainstream, it seems that many meat and dairy alternatives are being launched every month, one more delicious than the other. Today, Vegans can treat themselves to incredibly realistic plant-based burgers, sausages, mince, and nuggets, vegan yogurt, vegan ice cream, vegan butter, and a growing selection of tasty dairy-free cheeses. Now, be aware that these products should be considered occasional treats as they fall under the umbrella of "junk food." On the other side of the vegan nutrition spectrum, health-promoting plant-based milk, such as almond milk, soy milk, and oat milk, takes over the industry bit by bit and becomes the new normal for many. Head on over to your city's (or town's) local coffee shop and ask for dairy-free options – you'll be surprised at how popular they have become.

Spices, oils, and herbs — Spices and herbs are what make a dish, and luckily for us, the vast majority of options are all inherently vegan-friendly. Vegetable oils like olive oil, avocado oil, and sunflower oil are all plant-based. Popular condiments like ketchup, hot sauce, soy sauce, vinegar, barbecue sauce, and tomato sauce are largely vegan-friendly as well – remember to check the ingredients label to be 100% sure of what you are buying. All types of natural herbs and spices, such as cumin, parsley, chili powder, rosemary, cinnamon, paprika, curry powder, cilantro, oregano, bay leaf, and countless others will bring your plant-based meals to the next level. There's no need for animals and animal products to make your dishes more appealing. Don't forget salt and pepper to taste too.

Do you now believe me when I say a vegan diet is far from bland, uninspired rabbit food? What's even better, in my opinion, is that all of these ingredients can be used in almost infinite combinations, so you are pretty much guaranteed never to get bored with what you're eating.

When considering all of these fantastic, diverse options, I am reminded of a famous quote from animal rights activist and philosopher Gary Francione:

"Veganism is not a sacrifice, it is a joy"

— GARY FRANCIONE

When we shift our mindset from restriction and deprivation to one of *abundance*, we can fully be ready to embark on our vegan journey without unnecessary fears or doubts.

TIME TO SHOP, WHAT TO LOOK FOR

It can be hard not to look like a lost child in the grocery store when you go for your first big shop as a vegan. While you now know what you can and can't eat, it can be quite tricky at first to turn your knowledge into a concrete list of meals or a fully-realized shopping list. That's why I encourage you to plan ahead of time and write down a week's worth of easy plant-based meals to get a good look at the staple ingredients you're going to need every week — fresh, frozen, packaged, and canned. To simplify this process for you, I decided to provide you with a week's worth of delicious meals in Chapter 5. Feel free to take a look at it before you head down to your local grocers.

Still, there are some plant-based staples that every vegan I know, myself included, will have on their weekly shopping list, essential items that should always be on hand in your kitchen – so, let's start with those.

You'll first stock up on bread or tortilla wraps, all-purpose flour, rice, oats, egg-free pasta, or noodles. These are crowd-pleasing, budget-friendly, widely accessible carbohydrate sources that will fill you up and make a complete meal paired with a protein source and healthy fats. Depending on how healthy you want your vegan diet to be, you might choose the whole grain option for each of these products – which as a nutritionist, I whole-heartedly encourage you to do.

Next, you want to make sure you have plenty of legumes in your cupboard for a reliable protein and fiber source. Buying dry beans and lentils will further stretch your dollar, but it will involve longer prepping and cooking times. Ultimately, the dry vs. canned choice will fall on what you value the most in your lifestyle – convenience or frugality. In terms of what legumes to buy, it all depends on your favorite meals. If you're a chili lover, you might want to stock up on black and kidney beans. If you love curries, then red lentils or chickpeas are going to be your legumes of choice. If you want to increase protein intake, make sure to pick up soybean products like firm tofu, edamame, TVP, and tempeh – they're not only incredibly healthy for you but also extremely versatile. Don't worry if you're unfamiliar with them or have no idea how to cook them yet, as I will go over the wonders of soybeans in the next chapter.

Vegetables and fruits should always be a part of your daily meal plan, so make sure to get your favorites on every shopping trip. I recommend you always include a generous amount of green leafy vegetables like spinach, kale, collards, or cabbage to get your recommended intake of essential vitamins and minerals. Highly versatile veggies like potatoes, carrots, and yams should also be on your weekly list of staples, as they can be incorporated into an endless combination of meals. You don't have to buy everything fresh if you're on a limited budget – frozen veggie mixes, frozen spinach, and peas, canned corn, or green beans are just as good as fresh, and the same goes for fruit. Along with crowd-pleasing staples like bananas and apples, make sure to pick up frozen berries for a powerful boost of antioxidants.

Now, move on to your nuts and seeds. These are much more convenient and budget-friendly when bought in bulk, and I suggest you focus on the more nutritionally dense varieties (like walnuts and almonds) and heart-healthy seeds like flax seeds and hemp seeds to get the most bang for your buck. Don't forget to pick up a tub of natural, sugar-free peanut butter for sandwiches, crackers, or a delicious oatmeal topping.

I would also recommend you stock up on a week's worth of non-dairy milk, whether it's soy milk, oat milk, almond, or cashew milk. You will end up using these non-dairy alternatives in all sorts of recipes, from pancakes to oatmeal and smoothies - not to mention the generous daily splash in your coffee or morning cereal. Plant milk is undoubtedly a staple.

Next, make sure you've got a well-stocked spice rack full of flavorful herbs, sauces, savory and sweet condiments. There's no limit with this one, but you may want to first focus on spices and herbs you're likely to use every day. Think garlic and onion powder, chili powder, Italian mix, curry powder, and maybe a good veggie stock to cover the basics. Add whatever else you like to these staples plus a good selection of versatile condiments like ketchup, soy sauce, hot sauce, mustard, or maple syrup — you'll be cooking flavorful, sumptuous vegan meals in no time. If looking to try something new and delicious, see if you can find some nutritional yeast (also known as "nooch") in your local health food store or at your regular big supermarket. These cheesy, savory flakes are a staple for many vegans, as they can provide a fair amount of vitamin B_{12} and other essential minerals in a tasty, cheese-like versatile condiment.

After you've got your plant-based staples sorted, it's time to pick up some treats and extras to make your diet that much more enjoyable. Start by heading over to your supermarket's frozen section and scouting the vegan options available, such as plant-based beef burgers, vegan chicken burgers, vegan sausages, nuggets, dairy-free ice cream, cheesecakes, and ready-meals. Some examples of beloved brands you might find are *Daiya, Beyond Meat, Impossible Foods, Gardein, Tofurky,* and *Morningstar Farms.* Check the chilled section for even more options like vegan-friendly cheeses, deli meats, yogurts, or head over to a health food store for a greater variety of products and brands. Many non-vegan brands, like ice cream giant Ben & Jerry's, offer plant-based versions of their classics (with more and more options coming out all the time, it seems).

Quite a few traditional junk food staples like frozen fries, hash browns, natural cereals, crackers, popcorn, and potato chips are already accidentally vegan. As long as you're checking each ingredient label thoroughly (more on this in Chapter 6), you can find plenty of vegan-friendly options in almost every grocery store aisle. Just arm yourself with a fair bit of patience, at least for your first time consciously shopping as a vegan, and see if some of your favorite snacks happen to be accidentally vegan already.

THE PERFECTLY BALANCED VEGAN PLATE

So, you've got your staple vegan foods ready (plus a few junk food items for comfort), and they are now replacing your old cupboard and fridge essentials. Do you know how to put them together to meet all your nutritional requirements and satisfy your taste buds? Depending on what your diet previously looked like or where you're from, answers may vary.

In a way, you have to go "back to school" and re-learn what a healthy plate looks like, according to the vegan food pyramid. The most straightforward manner of looking at this nutritional eating guideline is to imagine a dish consisting of 50% vegetables and fruits, 25% whole grains, and 25% plant-based protein.[1] Of course, this meal type doesn't strictly have to be on a plate or be 100% faithful to these percentages. What this guideline can do, however, is provide you with a great blueprint to keep in mind when preparing a meal or shopping for new ingredients.

As long as you do your best to get as close to this model plate as you can, you will be doing your body a favor.

What would a balanced plate like this look like in practical terms? A great example would be a tasty plant-based wrap: you've got your whole wheat or corn tortilla, a filling of spicy kidney beans or black beans, and a whole lot of lettuce, spinach, sweetcorn, tomatoes, onions, and avocado slices to bulk up the veggie percentage. This simple meal is not only filling and delicious but also incredibly healthy and quick to make. A win-win all around.

Another perfect example of a balanced vegan plate is a classic Buddha Bowl: a whole food bowl packed with a mix of green leafy vegetables and root vegetables, a whole grain of your choice (like quinoa or brown rice), and a portion of beans, like chickpeas or hummus. I like adding a sprinkle of sunflower seeds on top of my lunch bowls too. This dish is endlessly customizable, incredibly fiber and nutrient-rich, and you guessed it – extremely easy and quick to prepare.

So, have you spotted a trend yet?

All the best plant-based, healthy dishes tend to be easy to make, requiring very little prep and cooking time. Cooking in bulk and meal prepping for the week can be sustainable, especially for new vegans. Making one big pot of minestrone, bean chili, lentil soup, or sweet potato and chickpea stew can last you for days – while requiring no more than 30 minutes to prepare.

So, to recap, here are the basics for creating a healthy and delicious vegan meal, every time: make vegetables the star of your meal, include whole grains and plant-based protein sources with every dish, and finally, swap or try new ingredients regularly – your vegan diet should be healthy, convenient, and always exciting!

VEGAN NUTRITION 101

So, what is the balanced vegan plate based off?

Before you get your chef's hat on and start experimenting with your plant-based diet, you should make sure you're aware of all your nutritional requirements as a vegan and how to safely get the necessary vitamins and minerals so that your body thrives. Let's start this off by covering the very basics of nutrition: macronutrients vs. micronutrients.

Macronutrients (sometimes shortened to "macros") refer to any diet building blocks: carbs, protein, and fat. On the other hand, micronutrients (sometimes referred to as "micros") are everything else your body needs to function: minerals and vitamins.

Carbs are the staple of every diet, including a vegan one. While they are our preferred source of glucose (our most important energy source), it can be effortless for us vegans to get more than we need, and that's why adding a good source of protein and fat in each meal is crucial to achieve a balanced diet.

Speaking of protein — how much do we need for our bodies to thrive? The RDA recommends an intake of 0.36 grams of protein daily for each pound of our body weight or 0.8 grams per kilogram of body weight.[2] This minimum protein intake works out as 15% of your total calories for the day in simpler terms. Despite the myth of vegan protein being "incomplete" or somewhat inferior to animal-based protein, the nutritional recommendations remain the same for meat-eaters and vegans. Any protein amount between 15% and 25% of your daily total calorie intake will ensure your body is well cared for.

Finally, fats are another essential macronutrient needed to feel full and satisfied, regulating our blood flow, hormone levels, and aiding in the absorption of essential vitamins.

Vegetables, nuts, and seeds should be your primary source of micronutrients, covering most of your nutritional needs when consumed daily. The good news is that vegans tend to get more of some essential vitamins than the average person following an omnivorous diet. Vegan diets can be naturally high in potassium, magnesium, vitamin C, vitamin E, vitamin A, and vitamin K.[3] The not so great news is that some other vitamins and minerals might be harder to get on a vegan diet, often requiring supplementation.

Vitamin B_{12} is the only vitamin vegans can't get from vegan food alone, so it has to be consumed through fortified foods (such as nut milk and nutritional yeast), or even better through convenient B_{12} supplements, available at any pharmacy or health store.

Vitamin B_{12} serves a crucial purpose in maintaining a healthy neurological function, aiding in red blood cell production, and creating and regulating DNA. Severe B_{12} deficiency carries a risk of irreversible damage to the brain and nervous system and less severe symptoms like fatigue and memory problems.[4] This vitamin can stay in our systems for up to four years, so, likely, most people going vegan for the first time won't experience any deficiency symptoms for a long time after transitioning and not supplementing. But this doesn't mean you don't have to start supplementing B_{12} straight away. It's recommended that vegans and non-vegans alike supplement this essential vitamin on top of their diet – yes, even a meat-heavy diet, since the soil through which our ancestors used to get their dose of B_{12} has become depleted through modern agricultural practices.[5]

Another essential vitamin that all of us, regardless of diet, should supplement is vitamin D. Its primary source is the same for vegans and non-vegans: sunshine. So if you don't catch enough rays throughout the year, make sure to supplement daily. The D cluster of vitamins promotes calcium absorption, regulates bone growth, and plays a vital role in stimulating immune function. Rich dietary sources are rare, and although most meat-eaters aim to get an adequate vitamin D intake from fatty fish, egg yolks, and butter, vitamin D is one of the most common nutrients to be found in fortified foods like cereal and milk. Note that vitamin D_3 is almost always derived from animals, while vitamin D_2 is plant-based and found in some varieties of mushrooms and fortified plant foods like nut milk or vegan breakfast cereal.

Iodine is another essential nutrient neglected too often. While non-vegans will typically get it from eating fish, vegans can get this one from seaweed or use iodized salt for cooking, which can be very convenient. Supplementing iodine will always be the most suitable option if you want to get enough.

Finally, we have omega-3 fatty acids. They are a crucial component of your body's cells, playing an essential role in your endocrine system (regulating hormones), immune system, and respiratory function. These essential nutrients are most commonly found in fatty fish and fish oil and some plant-based foods like flaxseed and canola oil. While it is possible to get enough omega-3 fatty acids from these plant foods alone, the reason why they might be so hard to get on a vegan diet is that the amount of omega-6 fatty acids found in most vegan diets greatly surpasses the amount of omega-3.

To get an adequate intake of omega-3, the optimal ratio of omega-6 to omega-3 must be 4:1 or less.[6] As most Western diets feature a much higher amount of omega-6 than recommended (around 16:1), this distorted ratio carries a risk of deficiency associated with fatigue, joint pain, cardiovascular issues, and menstrual problems in women. So, unless you're ready and willing to give up health-promoting, delicious omega-6 containing foods like avocados, sesame seeds and tahini, walnuts, and tofu, supplementation will again be your best bet.

As a nutritionist, I can safely say that everybody should supplement crucial nutrients daily regardless of their diet. Still, it is incredibly vital for those new to veganism to make sure they are regularly supplementing, as removing your usual sources of these vitamins might lead to unwanted health problems down the road.

So, how can you make sure you are nourishing your body as you should?

Following the balanced plate, the guideline is the first step in recognizing what ratio of macros to micros to include in your meals. Using an online nutrition calculator like *Cronometer* is a great way to ensure your body is getting what it needs. I would also recommend downloading Dr. Michael Greger's *Daily Dozen* app for optimizing your whole food intake. Even though it's delicious, vegan junk food should always be consumed in moderation. Vegan cheese, chips, chocolate, and plant-based burgers are generally very high in saturated fat, refined sugar, and sodium – while providing very little nutritional value.

I realize this may all sound very boring to you, but being conscious of your dietary requirements is vital when transitioning to veganism, as you may not be used to tracking your daily nutrients and calorie intake. Furthermore, a lot of people will often not eat enough when going vegan. You want to avoid this altogether – let's face it, fatigue doesn't make for a happy (let alone healthy) vegan or for an inspirational role model to look up to. You won't have to keep tracking your meals forever, though. A couple of weeks will be enough for you to figure out what you should be eating intuitively.

When planned appropriately and consciously, a whole food vegan diet will give you the best energy, mental focus, and mood of your life. There is absolutely no sense in taking unnecessary risks when it comes to nutrition – especially when your meals don't sacrifice incredible taste for the sake of optimal health!

5

YOUR EASY FIRST
PLANT-BASED WEEK

*Y*ou might be having trouble picturing what a delicious, healthful, and 100% plant-based dish could look like, especially if you're keen to keep track of your macros and micros intake. I can promise you that all those guidelines will get more natural and more intuitive to follow as time goes on and that you will learn to listen to your body on a vegan diet the same way you were used to on a standard diet.

When you start with veganism, you may feel hungrier, as plant-based foods generally don't contain as many calories as animal products. You might also have trouble getting enough calories because of an increased sense of fullness, thanks to a higher fiber content than what you may be used to. Both of these scenarios are completely fine, as long as you know what's happening with your new plant-fueled body.

You may find yourself missing certain flavors, like cheese or meat, which is perfectly normal. Remember that you are breaking the habits of a lifetime, so allow a generous adjustment period to find new flavors to love and ingenious vegan substitutes to replace the dishes you enjoy the most.

Experimenting with new ingredients and finding healthy vegan versions of your favorite flavors can help you curb those cravings – but you likely have no idea where to start. That's why I have compiled some of my favorite vegan dishes to inspire and motivate you to get cooking throughout your first vegan week. You might not enjoy the sound of all of them, but I can guarantee you'll be able to find something you love in the mix – remember to keep an open mind, and you may be surprised at how tasty and easy to make these healthy, plant-based recipes can be.

ENERGIZING BREAKFASTS

Some people enjoy savory breakfasts, while others like to indulge in their sweet tooth first thing in the morning, and the good news is that there are plenty of exciting vegan recipes for both of these camps.

Loaded Oatmeal — A classic bowl of oatmeal is an excellent option for the more health-conscious who like to keep their meals under budget. Take one half a cup of quick oats with your choice of plant milk. Cook it on the stovetop on low heat until thickened. Top it all off with fresh or dried fruit (banana coins, blueberries, and raisins are my personal favorite), walnuts or almond pieces, and a mix of hemp seeds and sunflower seeds – it will keep you full until lunchtime. If you need your oatmeal on the sweeter side, a drizzle of maple syrup or agave syrup will go a long way. One more tip, cinnamon can make it taste even more comforting.

Tofu Scramble — This breakfast scramble is the perfect choice for those who used to love eggs in the morning and have a little extra time to cook in the early hours. You're going to need extra firm tofu for this (it can be found in all Asian super-markets and health food stores), making sure to squeeze all the water out with your hands before adding it to the pan.

Start by pan-frying some onions, garlic, peppers, spinach, and mushrooms, before carefully crumbling the squeezed tofu into the pan. This soy product is relatively flavorless by nature, but it can soak up and retain all the flavors and spices it's cooked with – so don't skimp on the seasoning. I like adding paprika, turmeric, cumin, salt, and pepper, plus a generous sprinkle of nutritional yeast for a delicious cheesy flavor. Add these spices in amounts to your liking. I prefer only a dash of turmeric, but more pepper and paprika, for example. Cook all the ingredients together until the tofu changes color and all the vegetables are thoroughly done. Serve piping hot, and maybe with a slice of whole-grain toast.

Plant-based Breakfast Burrito — This is another savory, protein-packed breakfast that will keep you full for hours, ideal for growing and hungry teenagers. Start by pan-frying onions and garlic on medium heat before adding a portion of spinach, cherry tomatoes, and a cup of potato chunks, seasoning with paprika, chili flakes, cumin, parsley, nutritional yeast, salt, and pepper.

Add half a cup of canned kidney or black beans as the potatoes soften, drain them from the can, and wash them in cold water beforehand. For the final step, fill a wholewheat or corn tortilla with your fried veggies and beans, and enjoy.

Classic Vegan Pancakes — Pancakes are a once in a while treat for me as they are certainly far from being whole foods, high in sugar, and relatively low on the nutritional side of a health-promoting vegan diet. However, to show you that you can still have all your favorite sweet treats as a vegan, I will share a recipe that will wow all your meat-eating friends – they taste just like classic pancakes.

In your mixing bowl, combine one cup of self-rising flour, two tablespoons of brown sugar, one tablespoon of baking powder, and a pinch of cinnamon and salt with one cup of plant milk, one tablespoon of apple cider vinegar or lemon juice, and a teaspoon of vanilla essence. Make the batter by the spoonful on low heat, flipping the pancake once the top and sides stop bubbling. Top your stack with maple syrup, fresh blueberries, and a spoonful of natural peanut butter – trust me, these will soon become a favorite for the whole family.

Green and Sweet Protein Smoothie — This is a staple smoothie for me - fresh, nutritious, and naturally sweet, it helps me get all the vitamins and minerals I need in one go. Like oatmeal bowls, Smoothies are endlessly customizable, so you can try different ingredient combinations every day and avoid getting bored. The only equipment you're going to need is a good, sturdy blender. A Vitamix is a top favorite among smoothie makers, but you can still have a delicious blend with a more affordable option. Use the one you have and blend for longer, or you can purchase one that's more within your budget.

My go-to green smoothie is made with two ripe bananas, a cup of frozen mixed berries, a cup of fresh spinach and kale, and a scoop of vegan vanilla protein powder, blended with a mix of ice cubes, water, and soy milk. Investing in a quality plant-based protein powder will ensure that your protein intake is optimal, without overloading beans and tofu, though it's not entirely necessary. Some brands I'd recommend are *Sunwarrior Protein, Raw Sports, Garden of Life,* and *Vivo Life.*

LUNCH MUNCHIES

When lunchtime comes around, I tend to look for speedy meals that will give me sustained energy throughout the afternoon, healthy options that won't weigh me down or lull me into the dreaded afternoon slump. The following are incredibly tasty lunch ideas that can be easily packed on-the-go and quickly prepared the night before.

Quinoa Buddha Bowl — I genuinely believe Buddha bowls are a cheat sheet for getting all your macros and micros in one tasty, fresh, and hearty meal. You can always mix them up using different ingredients and dressings, so you can get the variety you need to make your diet as exciting as it can be. Quinoa Buddha bowls are some of my favorites, as using quinoa as the base of your bowl can help you get more plant-based protein in.

Following the balanced plate ratio, fill half your bowl with plenty of vegetables, like steamed kale, roasted broccoli, or pan-fried collard greens. Your cooked quinoa, or any whole grain you prefer, will take 25% of your plate, with your choice of chickpeas, beans, tofu, or tempeh (another protein-packed soybean product usually stocked in Asian food stores) as the remaining 25%. Be sure to add a delicious dressing to comple-ment all the ingredients, like some mashed avocado with garlic and chili flakes, a cheesy homemade sauce with blended cashews and nutritional yeast, or even a simple soy sauce and vinegar mix.

Peanut Sauce Stir-fry — This is another simple dish that is incredibly easy to customize. It's also a superb recipe for using up leftover vegetables in a tasty, healthy way. To start, pan-fry garlic and onions in a pan before adding your choice of vegetables (I recommend snap peas, soybean sprouts, cabbage, and carrots for the best crunch) and a generous drizzle of soy sauce and white vinegar. For your protein, choose between extra firm tofu, tempeh, or seitan (a protein-packed wheat product with a convenient meaty texture) to fry alongside your vegetables.

Allow 15 minutes for all the ingredients to cook evenly, and while you're waiting by the stove, start preparing the real star of this meal: the spicy, sweet peanut sauce. To make this sauce, mix two tablespoons of natural peanut butter with one table-spoon of soy sauce, a teaspoon of vinegar, a tablespoon of maple syrup, and a good sprinkle of chili flakes and garlic powder. Now mix all of the ingredients with a spoon or fork until smooth. Then, pour the sauce over your stir-fry – you're going to crave this daily.

Quick and Easy Chickpea Wrap — This is a fresh, healthy wrap recipe that requires a minimal amount of cooking, perfect for those busy days.

The cooking part of the process is very straightforward: all you need to do is pan-fry a can of chickpeas with onions, garlic, cumin, and parsley, just enough to coat the chickpeas in all those rich flavors. Next, spread some mashed avocado or hummus on whole wheat or corn tortilla, add the cooked chick-peas, romaine lettuce or baby spinach, sweet pepper slices, and cucumber strips. Roll up your wrap and enjoy on your lunch break.

Foolproof Pasta Salad — Fortunately for all you pasta lovers out there, whole wheat pasta makes for a delicious, hearty, and healthy alternative to your regular spaghetti. One of my favorite ways to enjoy a good bowl of pasta is making a fresh and colorful pasta salad, ideal for packing on-the-go.

Cook a portion of short pasta (such as penne) as instructed on the package, and leave it to cool for several minutes once drained. Next, prepare a base with your choices of leafy greens, such as baby spinach, romaine lettuce, or arugula, and add your protein source – chickpeas, seitan, butter beans, lima beans work perfectly with this dish. Add your chilled pasta into the mix and prepare a delicious dressing to bring it all together. Nothing beats a simple olive oil, garlic, rosemary, oregano, and black olives finish. Feel free to add whatever you'd like to this simple recipe: sweetcorn, baby tomatoes, peppers, avocado slices... there is no limit to the nutritious vegetables you can use – make sure you chill your pasta salad in the fridge first.

GO-TO COMFORT DINNERS

Dinnertime is a time of relaxation for me when I can unwind and take it slow. That's why I love making big pots of delicious, comforting plant-based food for the whole family that can be stored for days in the fridge, so I always have something to turn to when getting home exhausted after a long day out.

Cozy Bean Chili — Nothing says dinnertime comfort like a hearty bean chili. I like to start by browning some onions and garlic in a big pot and adding enough tomato sauce to cover them. Next, add your favorite mix of beans (kidney beans, lima beans, and black beans are my ideal combination) and plenty of cumin, smoked paprika, black pepper, salt, parsley, cilantro, and of course, chili powder. Let the chili simmer for 20 minutes, add spinach, frozen peas, and corn as it starts thickening up – a dash of nutritional yeast on top (before serving) can take it to the next level.

This soup will taste even better the following day, so make sure to save some (if you can, that is).

Creamy Chickpea Curry — This simple curry recipe has quickly become a staple for my family. It isn't hard to see why though, as it's unbelievably quick and easy to prepare, it's incredibly nutritious, and packed with flavor!

You want to start by boiling a cup of basmati rice to cook alongside your curry, ultimately taking you 15 minutes max. After frying onions and garlic in a pan, add a generous amount of curry powder, cumin, paprika, parsley, mustard seeds, and turmeric before covering the vegetables with tomato sauce. Add in a can of chickpeas to the sauce, and let it all simmer for about 10 minutes – the final step is adding a good splash of your favorite plant milk for extra creaminess. Your rice will be done by now, so fluff it up with a fork before serving alongside your chickpea curry, and make sure you leave enough for seconds.

Mediterranean Lentil Soup — Green lentils are a nutritional powerhouse, providing you with plenty of fiber, iron, and zinc. They cook quicker when soaked for a couple of hours in cold water, bringing the total cooking time to around 30 minutes only. Once the lentils are washed and drained, add a large clove of garlic, vegetable stock, celery, tomato sauce, cumin, parsley, and a squeeze of lemon juice to the pot. You can also add some peeled potato chunks to the mix and some spinach or kale for a heartier soup.

Cover with just enough water and let the soup simmer on medium heat for at least 30 minutes, regularly checking as lentils tend to absorb much of the boiling water. Sprinkle a bit of salt and pepper at the very end of the cooking process, and serve with your favorite vegan-friendly bread roll.

Cheeseless Mac and Cheese — This is undoubtedly a home run with the kids. The cheesy, savory taste and creaminess of your traditional mac and cheese are all there but reimagined in a dairy-free, healthy vegan dinner.

Cook the macaroni as the package instructs while preparing your cheesy vegan sauce. This sauce's key ingredient is a cup of unsalted cashews, ideally soaked overnight or even for a couple of hours. Add them to a blender along with ½ cup of your choice of plant milk and a very generous helping of nutritional yeast (that's the secret ingredient for perfect plant-based cheesiness).

Once blended and smooth, put the mixture aside before frying a couple of minced garlic cloves on medium heat. Add your choice of vegetables (frozen peas are always one of the most popular options) to the pan and pour your cheesy cashew sauce in, stirring well. Now, it's time to drain your mac and add it to the bubbling sauce. Simmer all the ingredients over low heat and add two tablespoons of lemon juice, one teaspoon of Dijon mustard, salt, and pepper – when your veggies are thoroughly cooked, you'll know your mac and cheese is ready.

I like adding some fresh parsley as I'm serving, but knowing just how delicious and comforting this recipe is, you'll probably want to dig right in.

Roasted Sweet Potato and Carrot Soup — This is a perfect soup for fall and winter, guaranteed to have you feeling right at the end of a hard day.

To start your soup, roast two large sweet potatoes and 200g of carrots for 30 minutes at 200C – just enough to release their natural sweetness. While your vegetables are in the oven, chop up onions and garlic to pan-fry with some olive oil, adding a cup of boiled water and vegetable stock once they have started softening. Add two medium-sized white potatoes, cut into small chunks, and start cooking them on medium heat along with your roasted sweet potatoes and carrots. Add rosemary, smoked paprika, salt, and pepper, and let it all simmer for 25 minutes, blending everything with a stick blender if needed.

When serving, I love sprinkling a generous amount of hemp seeds on top to boost this soup's nutritional value and add a hearty, satisfying crunch.

6

WHAT TO WATCH OUT FOR

*T*his could be a hard truth for you: no one can be 100% vegan through and through.

Striving for perfection on a vegan lifestyle is a recipe for disaster, as there are some non-vegan items and processes you can't avoid when living in a meat-eating world, from the leather seats of a car to the animal by-products used in conventional medications. Remember that being informed and always making an effort to do your best make you an ethical vegan – nothing else.

Carefully reading labels is not something most of us are used to, especially if we are not the health-conscious or perpetual dieter type. Your first shopping trip as a vegan will likely have you flipping over packages and bottles, thoroughly reading ingredients labels for any indication of animal products. But what exactly should you be looking for? A carton of milk is a carton of milk, a steak is a steak, and fish sticks are fish sticks, but what about the more subtle, hidden animal products that feature in many of your favorite snacks, toiletries, and processed foods?

This chapter will help you identify some of the most common non-vegan items while adjusting to this new lifestyle. It might take a little while to learn how to read labels and identify sneaky animal products, so be kind to yourself by taking the time to learn from your mistakes, move forward, and do better the next time. You've got this!

ANIMAL FATS AND SCRAPS

You might very well be surprised by the number of everyday products that contain different types of animal fats and secretions. As with many other animal by-products in this list, you'll find that these ingredients are incredibly hard to read and pronounce, giving you little to no indication of them.

Gelatin is one of the most common animal ingredients found in popular candy, cosmetics, or even as a fining agent for clearing wines. Gelatin is a cheap, glue-like substance obtained by boiling skin, tendons, horns, ligaments, or bones of animals with water (usually cows or pigs). It is one of the most available thickeners for companies to use in their products. It combines all the meat industry's leftovers in a flavorless, colorless, and versatile gel substance.

You'll find gelatin in some fruit jams, gummy candy, marshmallows, fruit gelatins and puddings, candy corn, and many other candy types. Gelatin is also used in several shampoo brands, cosmetic creams, face masks, nail treatments, and a standard coating for capsules, pills, and even photographic film. It's quite fortunate that the world has moved mostly to digital pictures now.

Lanolin is another pervasive product in the food and cosmetic industries. It is a greasy, fatty built-up substance taken from sheep's wool, used in several moisturizers, lipsticks, makeup removers, and other skincare products to help achieve a smooth, soft appearance. If you're thinking *eeew* already, I've got some bad news for you: Lanolin has been hiding in your breakfast cereal this whole time. Lanolin is used in many popular cereal brands as a vitamin D supplement and features as an emollient in chewing gum types.

Glycerin, also known as *glycerol*, is a liquid with a sweet taste derived from plant oils and animal fat (mostly beef tallow). It can be found in makeup products, hair gel, mouthwash, chewing gum, toothpaste, soap, and some food items like cookies, ice cream, or other dessert products. Not all brands will specify if their glycerol is plant-based or tallow based, so if you come across this ingredient during your shopping, you'll have to do more extensive research.

Stearic acid is another common additive in some plastic bags, vitamin supplements, and toiletries (especially shampoo and soap) — just like with glycerin, it is not always easy to tell whether it's vegan or not. Stearic acid is a fatty acid used to stabilize various finished products and avoid separation (for example, in some peanut butter or margarine brands). It can either be made from vegetable oils, like palm oil or from animal fats. It is typically made from a mix of the two, but many manufacturers won't disclose its exact origin.

Finally, we have **keratin**, a rather popular ingredient in various hair care products and treatments. It is a structural protein derived from the meat industry's scraps, including hooves, feathers, animal hair, and horns. Now, that's something I definitely wouldn't want to put in my hair, no matter how shiny it's going to make it look.

INSECT INGREDIENTS

Yes, I know what you're thinking. Oddly enough, specific types of insects are routinely used in the food and cosmetic industries to obtain dyes, add shine, or increase moisture.

If you've ever bought red lipstick or eaten red candy, you have probably already encountered **carmine**. This natural red dye is collected by crushing a South American beetle, the cochineal scale. This industry's history spans millennia: when the Spanish invaded Mexico in the early 1500s, they were astonished by the bright red color found in local textiles. Back in Europe, red was one of the most challenging pigments to obtain. Fast-forward a few years, and cochineal would become the second-largest export of the New World, and its popularity still hasn't waned in the modern-day.[1] Manufacturers rarely label carmine as such in their products' ingredients, so watch out for the not-so-secret codes **E120** and **Natural Red 4** when picking up vibrant red products such as fruit drinks, sodas, candy, syrups, and red-colored makeup items.

Snail slime (yes, the sticky substance oozing out of snails as they move) is also frequently used in anti-aging creams and face masks, under the scientific name of *helix aspersa muller glyco-conjugates* – which is quite catchy if you ask me.

Lac bug secretions, labeled as **shellac**, are also routinely used in hair sprays, eyeliners, and mascaras to stimulate hydrating and moisturizing properties. You'll come across this product under the name of *confectioner's glaze* in the food industry, the ingredient giving some popular candy its appealing sheen.

EGG BY-PRODUCTS

You may also risk purchasing eggs without realizing it if you quite don't know what to look for. **Albumen**, most commonly known as egg white, can be found in skincare products like face masks and in popular food products like baked goods, or as a clarifying agent in beers and wines. There are also several cocktails featuring egg white as one of their main ingredients, so stay clear of foamy cocktails like *Whiskey Sour, White Lady, Vodka Sour, Gin Fizz,* and *Clover Club.*

Egg wash, a liquid obtained by beating eggs, is commonly found in pastries like croissants, scones, pretzels, or breaded food products. Egg by-products will usually appear in bold when listed on the packaging, as eggs are possibly dangerous, common allergens, but they can be hard to spot when purchasing loose baked goods. In this case, the best course of action is asking the baker, keeping in mind that glossy-looking pastries will more likely than not contain egg wash.

ANIMAL BONES AND FISH BLADDERS

You won't find actual bones in your food and drink (we can all imagine the lawsuits if that were ever the case), but if you live in the United States, there's a huge chance you've been consuming products filtered through animal bones all along.

White sugar is the perfect example of a seemingly animal-free product that may have bone filtration within its production process. Filtering raw cane sugar through ground bones (**bone char**) is an old manufacturing tradition that has fallen out of style in most of Europe and Oceania. However, it's still very much in use in the United States and Asia.[2] This is how white sugar is produced, the same white sugar that goes into thousands of pastries, sodas, granola bars, and desserts – making it virtually impossible to know whether a processed product is entirely vegan. That's where the vegan-friendly stamp you might have seen on some packaged products comes in handy – sometimes, it's either that or contacting the manufacturer yourself, and the majority of us certainly don't have time for that. Bone char may also be found in some tattoo ink brands, which could contain animal glycerin, shellac, and gelatin – so make sure you ask your tattoo artist about where their ink comes from if you're planning to get something done, it will stay on your body forever.

You should also be aware that filtering or clarifying products through animal parts is not exclusive to white sugar. *Isinglass*, for example, a substance made from dried fish bladders, is used as a fining agent in some beers (like British real ales), wines, and collagen in fruit jellies and jelly puddings.

MILK AND OTHER DAIRY INGREDIENTS

Milk is everywhere. Milk by-products have a sneaky way of finding themselves in many modest products, so checking the ingredients label will always be the only way of knowing what exactly is hiding in your food. I remember being baffled for a long time whenever I would turn a pack of potato chips around to find that they contain some milk derivative that I could never have tasted.

Casein (most notably found in Recaldent oral care products), a leftover protein of cheese production, can also be found in medicines and otherwise dairy-free products like baked goods, margarine, and coffee creamers. The more common **whey**, another cheese by-product, can be found in candy, bread, savory snacks like potato chips, dark chocolate, cereal bars, instant noodles, and protein powders (to name a few). Nine times out of ten, you'll find milk by-products listed as "**milk solids**" or "**milk traces**," a frustrating ordeal when these ingredients do nothing to improve or modify a product's flavor. Fortunately for us, dairy by-products will often be highlighted in bold on the ingredients list. They are widespread allergens – identifying them is much easier than spotting crushed beetles or tallow.

This chapter is far from being an extensive list. There is a virtually endless amount of sneaky (and quite unappetizing) animal products used in everyday items. To name a few more, you can find *ambergris* (whale vomit) in perfumes, *squalene* (shark liver oil) in deodorants, *musk oil* (genital secretions of deer, otters, or beavers) in fragrances and oils, and *guanine* (fish scales) in shimmery makeup products. The pervasiveness and subtleness of these products are why looking for a vegan-friendly logo on the packaging is crucial.

Unfortunately, not all brands have caught up with the times, so you may find entirely plant-based, cruelty-free products that have yet to be officially labeled. The best way to avoid purchasing animal product-laden items is by buying from reputable vegan-friendly brands. These brands will give your mind some peace when it comes to sticking to your beliefs and supporting ethical, like-minded businesses simultaneously. Cruelty-free, vegan-friendly brands are slowly becoming the new normal, so purchasing products from beauty brands like *E.l.f.* and *KVD Vegan Beauty*, rather than MAC or LÓreal, should be a breeze. On the other hand, where food products are concerned, you might want to use additional tools (on top of the good old checking labels routine) to identify whether a product is 100% vegan or not.

Note that you will undoubtedly come across a vague disclaimer found on all sorts of plant-based products throughout your label-checking journey: *"may contain traces of milk"* or *"may contain traces of eggs."* You'll be happy to know that the product in question is still vegan – just produced in a factory that handles dairy products or eggs, with a very slim chance of cross-contamination. It's required by law that manufacturers state this disclaimer on all packaging as the small chance of finding traces of dairy or eggs in a product may cause severe allergic reactions in some consumers.

I recommend checking the handy websites *isitvegan.net* or *doublecheckvegan.com* to confirm a product's vegan-friendliness further when in doubt and heading over to *barnivore.com* for double-checking your beers, wines, and liquors. This website is a trusted and fantastic directory for determining if an alcoholic drink is suitable for vegans, so you won't have to guess blindly, or even worse, ask a clueless bartender for answers.

Now, I understand that this may sound like a whole lot to remember, but keep in mind that checking the ingredients label of new products will only be a concern when looking to buy items you're not familiar with, so you'll likely only have to do it once or twice. You will soon identify the vegan-friendly products you love, incorporate them into your routine, and never have to read their ingredients list ever again.

7

VEGANISM IN PUBLIC

*B*eing a new vegan is much like being a chronic introvert — it's all fine and good until you have to get out of the house.

When I first went vegan, ditching all sorts of animal products from my diet and life, I found being vegan at home as easy as following any other diet. I haven't been a dieter myself, but I knew how to stay on track to ensure I got enough nutrition throughout the day. It's quite simple: if you only buy vegan groceries, you'll only have vegan food in your kitchen, and you'll only make vegan meals and snacks – no cheesy options, no second thoughts.

Then, I received an invite to a birthday party.

I must admit it was a nerve-wracking experience. The evening soon took a very stereotypical turn with me having no choice but to order a side salad (hold the eggs and the creamy dressing) and a portion of fries. Embarrassed and quite hungry, I left the party swearing I will be more prepared next time, so I could show my non-vegan friends just how delicious and satisfying a vegan diet could be.

And prepare, I did.

This chapter will lay out a game plan you can follow when going out to non-vegan restaurants and takeaway joints, eating on road trips, and traveling abroad. Let's not stick to boring side salads that ruin our evening out.

NAVIGATING RESTAURANT OPTIONS

Unless you're on your way to a vegan restaurant, you should not assume that all restaurants will cater to your dietary needs. Veganism has made significant strides in the last five years, so I'm well aware that many of the challenges I used to face back then when eating out won't apply as much anymore. Still, depending on where you live, your options will always be limited compared to what your non-vegan friends could have – but don't let that scare you.

The key to a successful, satisfying dinner out as a vegan is research. You should make sure to research the restaurant, bar, or pub you're visiting to preview their menu ahead of time. It will leave you more than enough time to prepare so you don't choke or get confused once the waiter comes for your order –

you want to avoid that sort of pressure at all costs. You shouldn't have any issues in today's world when looking up a place online, as it's highly unlikely your destination won't have any online presence.

Start by googling the restaurant's name, see what comes up, and head over to their website, Facebook page, Google business account, Yelp, or TripAdvisor listing. You'll undoubtedly find a menu and some helpful reviews when you leave no stone (or in this case, link) unturned. If you're fortunate, you might even discover several vegetarian and vegan options, often with a handy code (*V, Ve, Vg,* or similar) right next to the dish's name to make them more easily identifiable. Quite a few eateries nowadays will have at least one entirely plant-based option, which hopefully will be to your liking.

Another common scenario would be to come across a restaurant with no vegan options but offering a few veggie-friendly ones and several customizable sides. Take it as a chance to get creative and try planning a full meal out of the meatless options you can find. For example, you may ask to take out the cheese from a veggie patty burger or hold the dairy-based dressing of a whole grain salad, swapping the animal product ingredients for avocado, corn, rice, etc. other plant-based food they have on hand. Order a couple of sides like veggie antipasti, fries, or hummus. There's nothing wrong in asking for more bread rolls to fill you up either, as long as you're making sure the bread or breadsticks are vegan by asking staff beforehand.

After planning your meal around sides and swapping a few ingredients, you'll likely end up with a pretty satisfying meal. However, if looking for something more, or if there are no customizable options for you, your best bet will be to call up the restaurant before visiting and ask them to prepare a special vegan meal for you. Now, I know what you're thinking – you can't imagine putting yourself on the spot like that or being "such a bother" by requesting a special meal.

While it is an understandable concern, you have nothing to worry about: restaurants are used to dealing with customers with all sorts of dietary requirements, like celiacs and lactose intolerants. They'd much rather be prepared for you in advance instead of figuring everything out last minute. It's a win for both parties, and there's no reason to be shy, so call them up with any doubts or questions you may have regarding their menu and accommodations.

Now, let's take a little step back.

Even though it's important to know how to be prepared when visiting non-vegan joints, it goes without saying that the easiest and best way to make sure both you and your party enjoy yourself when eating out is to choose vegan or vegan-friendly spots. If you have followed most of my previous guidelines for a stress-free vegan transition, you have already taken a second look at your social circle and hopefully weed out the people who won't support your new lifestyle. Those who truly matter, those who empathize with your choice and care for your well-being won't have an issue with letting you take the lead when choosing where to eat. Logically speaking, it makes much more sense to have the person with special requirements have a say when that choice impacts them – non-vegans can easily eat and enjoy vegan food, but vegans cannot give up their beliefs and change their lifestyle for the comfort of others. You might find out that your support system will have a more pleasant time when they know you're comfortable and happy with the restaurant you're going to. They might discover new foods and flavors they didn't know existed and find new favorite dishes in the cuisine they least expected to find them in. Taking your family, friends, or partner to a vegan restaurant is a fantastic opportunity for you to show what your diet is all about. Down the line, it will likely be an enjoyable memory for everyone involved.

So, how can you find vegan or vegan-friendly joints that will wow both you and your meat-eating social circle?

The first place I recommend you head over to is *Happycow.net*, available as an app and a very user-friendly, beloved website. This online directory lists vegan and vegan-friendly restaurants, food trucks, takeaway joints, bakeries, and supermarkets worldwide. Happycow is, hands-down, a more thorough and extensive guide for restaurant-loving vegans, so no matter where you live, you can find something that will cater to your needs. The website features user reviews, pictures, full menus, price ranges, area maps, and overall brief descriptions of each eatery curated by real users. If you're passionate about your local vegan food, I suggest you create an account and become an active user. You'll be able to connect with local vegans, review your favorite and least favorite spots in town, and even suggest a new entry if you encounter an undiscovered vegan-friendly gem. Besides Happy-cow, I would recommend checking out other directories such as *Vegman.org*, *Vanilla-bean.com*, and the app VeganXpress. Note that even popular websites not catered explicitly to vegans like Yelp, TripAdvisor, and TimeOut will point out whether a restaurant is vegan-friendly or not as part of the description – a real sign that times are changing in our favor.

It's up to you to decide whether to go to a fully vegan restaurant or opt for a spot catering to all, with several great vegan options. As a last little tip, I encourage you to pay special attention to "ethnic" restaurants, which will more likely cater to your needs than an all-American or pan-European spot (except the odd Mediterranean or authentic Italian restaurant). International cuisines like Indian, Chinese, Ethiopian, Mexican, and Thai are well-known for their focus on plant-based ingredients. They will undoubtedly have much more variety for vegans to enjoy than your regular burger joint. Chinese, Thai, and Vietnamese restaurants will have plenty of tofu-based dishes to enjoy, along with noodles, fried rice, vegetable spring rolls, spicy vegetable curries, and even mock meat dishes. The Buddhist tradition all heavily influences these cuisines, so your server will likely be familiar with the idea of vegetarianism and veganism - make sure to ask if any eggs or fish sauce are lurking in your vegetarian stir-fry, and you're good to go. Indian cuisine, especially if South Indian, will often offer you the most variety: endless types of curries, dosas, onion bhajis, and samosas are just scratching the surface of how colorful and delicious vegan Indian food can be. Mexican food relies on many of the standard staples of a vegan diet. As long as you avoid cheese and sour cream, you can be sure to leave the eating spot full and satisfied with beans, rice, avocado, pico de gallo, guacamole, nacho chips, and corn tortillas. Ethiopian cuisine is one of my all-time favorites when going out. You can usually order a set meal based around injera bread (an addictively tasty savory pancake) and surrounded by delicious, hearty plant-based stews to share. The result is a healthy, filling meal packed with lentils, potatoes, and chickpeas, which is guaranteed to have something for everybody in the group to enjoy. Finally, Mediterranean cuisines like Italian, Greek, Israeli, and Lebanese can offer vegan options full of fresh flavors. They feature dips like hummus, olive tapenade, and baba ganoush along with fluffy pita bread and tomato-based pasta – all topped with a generous amount of heart-healthy olive oil. Picking a restaurant according to the vegan-friendliness of the featured cuisine is the best way to make sure you'll get your money's worth. No substitutions or dish-tweaking is necessary.

One important thing to be mindful of before you plan your night out is that accidents can and (more likely than not) happen in a non-vegan environment. Your "veganized" order might turn up in front of you with an egg on top, mayo on the side, or even a full-on piece of meat or fish. It might be a classic case of miscommunication, as not everyone will fully understand what you can and cannot eat, or just a genuine mistake on the part of the chef and waiter serving you. Whatever the case and however upsetting, the best way to deal with this situation is to remain calm, point out the mishap, and return the order untouched. The staff will likely be apologetic and do their best to correct the mistake by offering you another meal. There's no point in making a scene and have everybody feeling uncomfortable. Everyone can make mistakes, and it doesn't make you a bad vegan to accept a dish you thought was vegan only to realize that it wasn't. Mess ups are bound to happen, and they can serve as great opportunities to become more responsible and diligent when eating out. It's all part of the learning process – not just for you but also for everyone around you.

TRAVELING VEGAN IS POSSIBLE

Even though we all love to go on trips and explore, traveling can sometimes be a pretty stressful ordeal, and I'm saying that without adding any special diet requirements into the mix just yet.

What does that say about traveling as a vegan, then?

I might be presenting this challenge as way more dramatic than it is - once again, adequate preparation and research are all you truly need. A fun day trip or a weekend road trip are two perfect opportunities for putting your meal prep skills to the test. Most of us have relied on gas stations, fast-food joints, and roadside diners when on the road, but switching to nutritious, easy-to-pack vegan snacks and packed lunches won't be a challenge when you're already familiar with meal prepping (which you should be by now). Of course, you might be able to find some vegan food along the way, but I believe better safe than sorry is the way to go, especially if you're looking to make your trip more budget-friendly. So, before heading out on your adventure, get prepping.

Some of my favorite snacks to pack for a short trip are home-made bliss balls (made with gooey dates and nut pieces), granola bars, crackers, trail mixes, popcorn, and tortilla chips. You might also consider packing a tub of hummus or a few single, portable packets of nut butter to have alongside your crackers and rice cakes if you're confident you'll be able to finish them all without leaving them overnight. I prefer bringing dry, non-perishable food items with me, rather than fruit pieces or fresh veg since they don't need refrigeration and can be brought on planes and across borders. If you want to pack something more substantial for camping or an extended trip through rural areas, I suggest you invest in some quality containers and a handy travel cooler to keep your meals fresh and dry. There's nothing worse than a soggy wrap or an overheated, melting tub of guacamole. Your go-to packed lunches will likely be sandwiches or wraps, as they are quite filling and make great easy-to-store meals that can be prepared in a flash. A couple of classic peanut butter and jelly sandwiches, avocado wraps, or a bean burrito will do the trick just fine. If you're planning on camping or stopping for a picnic, consider bringing a big tub of guac to share, a creamy potato salad with vegan mayo, a pasta salad, a couscous bowl, or even some homemade baked goods like vegan brownies and oatmeal cookies. When you have a cooler, the sky's the limit. And remember that at any point during your trip, you can open the Happycow app and scout for hidden vegan-friendly gems in the area – it's always worth a try.

Even though I've had a fair share of prepping before weekend trips, making sure to pack at least two full meals for the road, I have to admit that I am not the biggest fan of meal prepping for trips. It's just a personal preference – between hotel bookings, gas stops, maps, and unforeseen obstacles, the last thing I want is to worry about preparing and packing tons of food for the road. Luckily, I have found that one big shopping trip to my favorite supermarket or health food store gets me everything that my family and I need for a couple of days. Some items include dried fruit, nuts, *Clif* bars, boxed grain salads, falafel, pasta salads, wraps, sandwiches, nut butter, savory snacks like pretzels and crackers, breadsticks, and chips. If I'm heading over to a campsite for the night, I also like stocking up on a few cans of vegan-friendly soups and stews that I can quickly heat for a warm, filling dinner. Whatever method serves best for you and your travel mates will ultimately be the winning one.

Traveling as a vegan can get a little more complicated when you're going abroad. The challenges pretty much start as soon as you board your flight, with all complimentary in-flight meals (beef or chicken?) being a no-go for vegans. Make sure to order a vegan meal ahead of time, which you can either do by visiting the airline's website or calling up customer service at least 48 hours before your flight. Don't forget to pack several snacks in your carrier bag too. Not all airlines will offer fully vegan meals, so if that's the case, make sure you have an adequate amount of food to keep you going while flying and for the first several hours after arriving at your destination. And speaking of that, ensure you have researched enough about its cuisine and food culture before you're heading to the airport – it will save you from a major headache once you're abroad with your phone data gone and an often sporadic Wi-Fi connection. Learn what you can about the country's staple dishes (how many are meat-heavy and how many are more veg-focused?). Make a list of vegan-friendly restaurants and supermarkets using Happycow or Vanilla Bean. If your destination's first language is different from your mother tongue, learn how to say "vegan" or explain what you can and cannot eat. Fortunately for the less language-savvy of us, there are quite a few resources out there that you can print or even save on your phone so that you can communicate your needs as a vegan to restaurant and hotel staff. I would personally recommend The Vegan Passport, an extensive vegan travel guide, and phrasebook created by The Vegan Society, which is available digitally and in paperback. The latest edition features the languages of over 96% of the world's population, so you are pretty much guaranteed to be covered wherever you go.

As someone who loves experiencing different cultures, I was initially taken back by the thought of never being able to taste the most beloved signature dishes of a foreign country again. But while it may be true that meat, fish, and all other animal products are often the backbone of most countries' cuisine, it doesn't mean you'll be missing out. For every meat-heavy main, there's usually a vegan side dish, traditional drink, or snack. Sampling everything a country's food has to offer may not be an option, but there will be plenty enough for you to try none-theless. When I decided to travel around East Asia and Southeast Asia after a full year of going vegan, I assumed I would be stuck eating bowls of unseasoned white rice the entire time. I thought I would be perpetually hungry and tempted by the non-vegan foods surrounding me.

Let me tell you — I've never been so glad to have been so, so wrong.

My journey through China, Thailand, Indonesia, and Vietnam was filled with delicious plant-based food: coconut curries, tofu stir-frys, mock meat dishes, noodles, and tempeh salads were available everywhere, and every single staff member I ended up speaking to had a good understanding of what veganism meant. I was also able to stumble across entirely vegetarian restaurants by just walking around; quiet, authentic eating spots offering many more vegan options than their American counterparts, always delicious and always incredibly budget-friendly. If traveling to any of these areas is your plan, look out for the international vegan restaurant chain Loving Hut. They offer an extensive menu of "veganized" traditional dishes at a wallet-friendly price – it's a great way to experience authentic foreign recipes without compromising your beliefs. You will also find that vegan and vegan-friendly restaurants are flourishing all over the world. So whether you're visiting Europe, Africa, South, or North America, know that you'll manage to find something for yourself – as long as you bring your Vegan Passport and Happycow app along for the ride.

To further expand on that, note that vegan-focused travel is also on the rise, with several new hotels and guesthouses offering an exclusively vegan menu to their guests – something you definitely wouldn't find in any other accommodation. I highly recommend stocking up on plant-based breakfast foods if a kitchen is not accessible during your stay, as regular hotels, hostels, and guesthouses are quite unlikely to have any vegan-friendly breakfast items in their buffets or menus. If the vegan-friendliness of your stay is essential to you, look no further than *vegan-welcome.com* or *veggie-hotels.com,* two excellent online directories listing all the vegan and vegan-friendly holiday accommodations available worldwide. *Vegvisits.com* is another valuable resource if you're keen to try homestays and house stays (think of it as a vegan Airbnb) with local vegans. This is a unique opportunity to experience your destination through the eyes of a local who will understand your lifestyle without any explanation, allowing you to sample homemade local dishes and get a real taste of what the vegan community looks like thousands of miles away from home. *Vegvisits* is a fairly new concept and website, with a small pool of members and listings, but with a lot of potential for authentic vegan community-building across borders. Wherever you end up visiting next during your vegan journey, I encourage you to connect with the vegans you're going to meet, whether they are accommodation hosts or restaurant staff, to nurture a sense of kinship and community. The world might feel more hostile and alien to you when first going vegan, but it's when vegans lift each other and create stable support systems among themselves that we can genuinely harness our power for change.

8

FROM EDUCATION TO ACTIVISM

"I'm an animal rights activist because I believe we won't have a planet if we continue to behave toward other species the way we do."

— JAMES CROMWELL

J have decided to create this guide as an introduction to the vegan diet and lifestyle, and however much in-depth this introduction aspires to be, it should not be taken as a complete guide to everything vegan. There will always be something more we can learn, many more topics to research, and many more pages I could write to explore how vegans worldwide lead their lives, their passions, and what aspects of veganism are still a hot topic up for debate. This chapter is all about growing into the vegan you aspire to be by deepening your knowledge, finding your community, or becoming a community leader – a vegan activist that other newcomers like you will perhaps look up to a few years down the line.

PLANT-BASED TO VEGAN: DEEPENING YOUR KNOWLEDGE

I have always believed in the power that education holds. Education is what combats ignorance, misinformation, and hate. At its core, veganism is a philosophy and a way of life, and like with any other philosophical belief; there is an almost infinite number of differing opinions and ongoing debates that make it a diverse movement. Your cultural background, country of origin, and social framework will impact how you see the world and the actions you take, so the kind of vegan you will become might also be profoundly influenced by these factors. As you continue your transition, you want to expand your knowledge about your lifestyle. Dive into different (and at times even contradictory) resources, and listen to the personal experience of other vegans fundamentally different from you in every way, so you can confront your biases and grow into a well-rounded, knowledgeable individual. During my life journey, I have learned that there is always something to unlearn, a new stone to turn, and then just when you thought you knew everything about a topic, a different insight can turn your world upside down in a matter of seconds. You will never know all that there is to know about veganism (I certainly don't either), but this doesn't mean that you shouldn't try your hardest to gather all the information available to you, so that you can craft your own set of beliefs and lifestyle practices.

Start by becoming more familiar with scientific studies related to a plant-based diet, so you can understand what research shows about the benefits of veganism. Let it inform you on how to lead a healthier lifestyle that will inspire those around you to give it a shot. There are several new nutritional studies and clinical trials coming out every year, so what you previously thought was law could completely change given a few years – make sure your information is up to date. When it comes to data and scientific evidence, social media can be either a blessing or a curse: sharing valuable information is now easier than ever, but it's also incredibly easy to misrepresent said information to an unsuspecting audience. If you familiarize yourself with how such studies are conducted, read and interpret data accurately, and spot biases or errors in existing studies, you can indeed be confident in your diet and challenge naysayers with your knowledge. Look for yearly and monthly roundups of the most critical studies on veganism on online publications like *Medium, PCRM, PlantBasedNews*, and *NutritionFacts.org*. Pinpointing these is the best way to stay updated on scientific news related to environmentalism and the vegan lifestyle, plant-based nutritional studies, and everything else in between.

Documentaries are also a great way of staying informed and diving deeper into specific topics related to veganism. Watching a movie is often much more comfortable and more accessible than reading a complex study, and it might be the best medium out there when trying to share eye-opening data and research with others. Watching a vegan documentary is what opened my eyes to the lifestyle in the first place. Some of the compelling documentaries I recommend you put on your watch list are *Earthlings* (which you can watch free of charge on the official website *nationearth.com*), *Cowspiracy, The Game Changers, Forks Over Knives, What The Health,* and *Dominion.* They are all available to watch on popular streaming services like Netflix, Amazon Prime, Hulu, and some even on Youtube. They cover a range of topics spanning climate change and the benefits of plant-based nutrition to the cruel practices and workings of the animal agriculture industry.

Next, find content creators to follow for a daily dose of inspiration. There are many YouTubers, Instagram influencers, or bloggers able to establish a personal connection with their audience and, in turn, spread the vegan message through a series of unique insights in a way that no documentary could ever achieve. Following these online personalities was a crucial step in my vegan journey. I was able to see what other vegans ate, thought, did with their time, and how they navigated the many challenges that I faced during the first few years of my transition. These were real people, not just anonymous accounts on a forum. So if you're anything like me and wish to find inspiring creators to guide you through your journey, I recommend you open your social media apps right now and get following. I'll mention some here that are not the ones I mentioned earlier. When it comes to vegan recipes and nutrition talk, I believe that *Caitlin Shoemaker, OhSheGlows, Bosh!, EdgyVeg, SweetPotatoSoul,* and the Buzzfeed-affiliated *Goodful* are some of the best voices in the vegan community. For everything fitness, look no further than *NaturallyStefanie,* and *Tess Begg.* If you're just on the lookout for entertaining vegan personalities, vloggers, and thoughtful opinion leaders, *Earthling Ed, Unnatural Vegan, Healthy Crazy Cool, BiteSizedVegan, High Carb Hannah,* and *Happy Healthy Vegan* are some of the most popular content creators worldwide.

Finally, I recommend you get yourself a couple of great books that delve deeper into different aspects of the vegan lifestyle and movement, covering many of the more controversial and sometimes misunderstood points of veganism. The following are all books I have purchased and thoroughly enjoyed myself, and the majority of them are still proudly displayed on my bookshelf and coffee table. Don't underestimate the power of gifting or lending a great read to a non-vegan friend either: I can count at least two people I "veganized" by letting them read one of my favorite vegan books. Dr. Michael Greger's, *How Not To Die* is a mainstream best-seller covering all the vegan nutrition bases.

Brenda Davis and Vesanto Melina's *Becoming Vegan* is the best guide to plant-based eating you'll ever find on the market. Marta Zaraska's *Meathooked* is a compelling deep-dive into our cultural obsession with eating meat. I would also recommend picking up Hal Herzog's *Some We Love, Some We Hate, Some We Eat,* and Jonathan Safran Foer's *Eating Animals* for two detailed explanations of the psychology behind our meat and animal products habit. Finally, Melanie Joy's *Why We Love Dogs, Eat Pigs, and Wear Cows* is a must-read for understanding "carnism," the default philosophy governing how we think about animals as a global culture.

CREATING YOUR COMMUNITY

You might have noticed that, throughout this guide, I've kept going back to the concept of community, stressing its importance in making your transition and overall life as a vegan as comfortable and as successful as it can be. That is because I've learned that having a reliable support system around you is fundamental to live as your authentic self. Having a supportive, like-minded community to turn to will give a sense of belonging, grounding you and allow for a space to talk about your unique struggles and achievements as a vegan without fear of judgment, mockery, or being misunderstood. Finding your community is the key to authentic growth as an individual, not only as a vegan – so, it's time to roll up your sleeves and find your place in the vegan movement.

As mentioned in earlier chapters, Facebook might be the most accessible place to start. You want to be looking for local vegan groups or vegan-focused events happening in your area to make some first connections. Try typing vegan + your city or country in the search bar and see what comes up. Introduce yourself, send a friend request or two, and if no particular event or meet-up is coming up anytime soon, why not take the lead and organize one yourself? It can be something simple like meeting for an oat milk latte at the only vegan-friendly coffee shop in town or checking out the best-rated vegan restaurant in the city with fellow first-timers. It's normal to be feeling shy in this kind of situation, but sometimes faking confidence can help us become genuinely more confident – so fight the insecurities and take the lead in setting up a small event if no one else has yet. Besides Facebook and Instagram, I recommend checking out *Meet-up.com* for vegan-related groups that might be meeting up in your area, or once again, creating a group yourself if you're not too happy with what you find. Creating a group is what I did after realizing my local one on Facebook was mostly inactive. Its few active members only posting recipes and sharing vegan news articles every few weeks, getting little to no engagement. So I decided to take the bull by the horns (in the most cruelty-free way possible, that is) and added all members individually before creating a little event to get together in real life. I picked a pretty random vegan-friendly restaurant I discovered through Happycow, set a time, and even asked for the members' phone numbers to create a chat for those interested. We talked almost every day during the week preceding the event, and by the time our little meet-up came around, we were far from total strangers. Fast-forward seven years later, and two of the people I met that evening are still some of my closest friends. Pretty impressive for an impromptu meet-up with a bunch of strangers from the internet, wouldn't you agree? Now, I'm not claiming that every connection you'll make will result in long-lasting, real friendships like these, but I can guarantee that meeting just one vegan in real life will make your first few months or even first year as a vegan much more manageable. You might live in a place where vegan events like food fairs, meet-ups, and educational talks happen every week, making it ten times easier to connect with like-minded people (and without having to organize anything yourself). However, you'll still have to make the first move if you're entirely new to the scene. Whether you're a natural extrovert or a socially-awkward introvert, remember that there are possibly a dozen other vegans who feel the same way you do: lost, shy, alone, but oh-so-eager to expand their worldview and meet new friends that will join them for the journey.

Volunteering for a vegan cause is another great way of making like-minded friends, and it is also one of the best ways to dedicate your free time to something meaningful, impactful for both the animals and the planet. You may want to try volunteering at an animal shelter or, better yet, look for an animal sanctuary near you to either visit or lend a helping hand. Animal sanctuaries are non-profit organizations offering life-long refuge to animals in need, most notably rescued farm animals like cows, pigs, and chickens. Another option worth researching is volunteering for or starting your own chapter of *Food Not Bombs*, an international collective providing free vegan and veggie food to others as a gesture of kindness and act of protest against world hunger and corruption. Participating in vegan-related initiatives like these will strengthen your connection to the local community and help you find like-minded, conscious vegans while contributing to making the world a better place. You might even realize that volunteering and organizing community events is something you love doing so much that you'll want to dedicate more of your time to causes you care for deeply. If that's the case, well then, you might want to give vegan activism a try. All vegans are somehow activists in their own right, even if they do not actively participate in demonstrations, direct action initiatives, politics, or advocacy. Vegans make an impact with every meal they prepare, every faux leather wallet they purchase, and every sandwich they ask staff to take the cheese off. But suppose you start finding yourself becoming more and more passionate about the lifestyle. In that case, it's only logical you will want the people around you, and ultimately the entire world, to go vegan as well. For their health, for the animals, for the environment.

So, what can you do to make a more significant impact and advocate for the ideas you believe in?

Leafleting is one of the oldest tricks in the book for vegan activists, and for a good reason: it allows space for passersby to approach you and ask questions about your cause if they are interested in what you have to say. Having them approach you limits any possible hostility and pressure for both parties. Upon joining this type of group for the day, you will usually be given several resources (pamphlets, guides, and vegan candy). You will be asked to give them out to passersby showing genuine interest in the vegan lifestyle while having a few talking points ready for all sorts of conversations on veganism. This form of activism is all about engaging the audience with your knowledge and passion for the vegan lifestyle, answering any questions they may have, and being both compassionate and persuasive in your replies. It's certainly not an easy task and not one you should take lightly if public speaking and confrontation are not your forte. No need to worry, though — if talking to strangers about veganism sounds like your worst nightmare come true, there are several other options available for a shy activist who's new to the game.

For example, you can try joining your local or nearest chapter of *Anonymous for the Voiceless*, an independent vegan organization operating internationally to raise public awareness of the cruelty of animal agriculture practices. The *AV* model is relatively straightforward and not that different from traditional leafleting: activists get together on scheduled dates to have meaningful conversations with the public about veganism while also showing the effects of animal agriculture on farm animals.

Activists will stand in the shape of a square, holding a laptop and wearing masks (hence the anonymous part) to draw passersby's attention while showing undercover footage of slaughterhouses and dairy farms. As more and more people stop to watch the footage shown, other activists, usually unmasked, will approach them to explain what they are seeing and discuss the concept of veganism, sharing their knowledge and experience of the lifestyle. What's great about this concept is you can either be a "conversationalist" or a laptop-holder, depending on your skills and which of the two you are most comfortable with. If you are passionate about spreading the message to the broader public but don't feel overly confident about speaking to (or often debating) with strangers about veganism, participating in this initiative as a laptop-holder might be the thing for you. Check if there is a group active in your area, and if there isn't, try reaching out to the organization first-hand at *anonymousforthevoiceless.org* to get the tools to get your group going.

I know that any form of activism involving public engagement may sound scary to a first-timer, but ultimately, it's the things that make us most uncomfortable that allow us to grow the most as people. Give it a try and take it as an opportunity to meet inspiring activists that will teach you the ropes. If you find out it's not your thing, know that there are many other forms of activism you can partake in. You can join or create a vegan/veggie society at your school or college, raise funds for animal charities and vegan advocacy groups, dedicate your social media platforms to spreading the vegan message, or even write a book or ebook like the one you are reading right now.

Everyone is different, and we all have a unique contribution to make to the world. You have a specific skill set and experience no one else has by just being you – what you choose to do with them is entirely up to you.

ANSWERING QUESTIONS YOU MAY HAVE

*I*f you're still with me so far, you've probably gained a thorough understanding of the vegan diet and lifestyle, how to transition to plant-based eating in the most stress-free way, and how to approach challenges you may encounter during your vegan journey.

And still, the burning questions keep coming.

Here, I will be addressing some of the most frequently asked questions newcomers might wonder about. To get a complete list of challenges and decisions that you might face down the road, you may need to dive deeper into the vegan world, but this is certainly somewhere to start if you find that there are still many doubts holding you back.

Will going vegan be hard to do?

When you see what's happening to animals, not at all. Going vegan will most certainly be a learning curve, but that doesn't necessarily mean it will be hard. In actuality, going vegan has never been as easy as it is now. As I discussed earlier, some people can transition to a vegan lifestyle overnight without any issues or unbearable cravings. For others, it might take months or sometimes even years to become fully vegan. What pace you'll go with is entirely up to you, so if you feel this is something you can get right into, drop all animal products overnight. Conversely, if you think you need more time to adjust, then take more time. There is no vegan police that will be checking in with you to make sure you've gone fully vegan after a set period, so take however long you need and use your *why power* to propel you forward each day.

There might be some aspects you will struggle with more, such as giving up cheese or switching to cruelty-free, vegan-friendly lifestyle products and clothing, but the best mindset to adopt is to think of these challenges as little obstacles along the way. Just follow the transition steps I have highlighted in Chapter three, and remember that the simplest things in life are rarely worth much – it's the challenges that allow us to grow and become the best versions of ourselves.

Will it be expensive?

Chances are you've heard the stereotype of the well-off, privileged vegan before. The truth that many newbies don't know is that anyone can easily be vegan on a budget. In fact, following a plant-based diet might even be more wallet-friendly than the lifestyle you are leading right now. Of course, the cost of your food depends on how you go about it. If everything you buy is pre-packaged, pre-cut, premium, and processed, plus you're eating out or getting takeaway most days of the week... well, you can expect to see a higher bill at the end of the month.

There is no need to go to Whole Foods (or any other high-end health food retailer) for your weekly shopping. Costco and non-membership grocery stores already have everything you need. Budget-friendly plant foods like canned or dry beans, lentils, rice and pasta, frozen vegetables, peanut butter, tofu, bananas, and oats can be the staples of your diet. They can be even more affordable when bought in bulk. As tasty as these are, you don't necessarily have to include meat or dairy replacements in your plant-based diet if your vegan burger obsession impacts your budget more than it should.

Give yourself time to learn how to make creative and delicious vegan meals at home using cheaper ingredients for an affordable and much healthier diet. The simple recipes I have included in this book revolve around many of the same elements for a reason: they can be incorporated in various dishes, and they can be used to create many plant-based food staples from scratch.

For example, the black beans you've grabbed in bulk can become delicious vegan burger patties. Making hummus from a can or two of chickpeas is incredibly budget-friendly, and the leftover water from the same can of chickpeas can be whipped into a "miracle" mayonnaise in a matter of minutes.

So, leave the fancy vegan restaurants for a special occasion, fill your cupboard with cheap and healthy plant-based staples, meal prep every week, and watch the savings grow.

Do I have to eat organic?

Not at all. Organic is not a requirement for veganism. Plant foods retain the same nutritional value, whether they are organic or not. Still, if you have come to veganism to become healthier and be more conscious about your food choices, buying mostly organic will benefit you significantly.

Those who want to limit the number of chemicals and pesticides in their food, without having to buy expensive organic fruits and vegetables every week, can check out the *"Dirty Dozen"* list created by the EWG (Environmental Working Group). This list changes every year, and it shows the top 12 products with the highest amount of pesticides – products you might want to eliminate from your diet entirely, or at least reduce if eating as organic as you can is essential to you. Alternatively, EWG also has a *"Clean 15"* list, containing the top 15 products with the lowest amount of pesticides found in them – perhaps your new staples.

Can I call myself vegan if I'm still buying animal products for clothing or personal care?

To make a complicated answer as straightforward as possible: no.

More recently, veganism has become synonymous with "plant-based," a dietary preference where all animal products are excluded from their diet, but not necessarily from their overall lifestyle. However, upon closer inspection of what the word "vegan" actually means, it's clear that veganism is an ethical and philosophical belief reaching far beyond diet alone. It's a lifestyle choice that seeks to exclude all animal exploitation from our clothing, furniture, beauty products, entertainment, etc.

In short, someone following a plant-based diet might eat the same foods that a vegan does (i.e., avoiding all animal products). Still, they do so as part of a usually short-term diet, merely striving to make healthier choices – this is unrelated to any philosophical belief. A plant-based eater might purchase cow leather or use makeup containing animal by-products, actions that vegans will always do their best to avoid. Suppose you have stopped eating animal products for a specific reason but have no intention of eliminating these products from your clothing or personal care items. In that case, you are technically not meeting the definition of veganism. If, however, your goal is to eliminate animal products from your life entirely, but you're just not there yet (as most seasoned vegans have been at some point), you could identify as a vegan – albeit one in transition.

I am allergic to soy. Where can I get vegan protein?

Any allergy or intolerance to plant-based foods will make your transition to veganism more challenging. Unfortunately, that's just the truth of it. Does that mean it'll be impossible or more challenging than you could manage? Not at all. Even in this specific case, having a soy allergy won't necessarily impact a vegan lifestyle's accessibility as much as you think it might. Although products like tofu, tempeh, soy milk, and meat substitutes like TVP are considered one of the best protein sources for plant-based eaters, they're by no means the only sources to rely on if concerned about your protein intake.

Seitan (a wheat by-product) is a high-protein healthy option for soy-avoidant vegans looking for a versatile, meaty texture to add to their meals. Quinoa and legumes like lentils, black beans, mung beans, peanuts, and chickpeas are also excellent protein sources. They are ones that can be easily incorporated into your diet daily. If you are looking for the most convenient option, a generous scoop of your favorite vegan protein powder will do – if just for a crazy busy day.

How do I handle friends or family that just don't get it?

As I previously discussed, you will likely be confronted by family members and friends who might want to debate with you, tease you for your choices, or repeatedly ask questions about your lifestyle. The constant stream of "where do you get your protein?" and "plants have feelings too!" can become nerve-grating, leaving you drained and hurt. On top of that, being around your family as they continue to eat animal products, especially around holidays, may be upsetting for you – it may even lead you to want to stop attending Thanksgiving and Christmas altogether.

Try to calm your mind and respectfully shut down questions and comments that upset you. Keep your *why power* in mind at all times. You know why veganism works for you, and you know why you want to be vegan — remember that. If being at the table becomes too much after a while, consider eating elsewhere or not attending these gatherings. There is no shame in wanting to nurture a more favorable environment for your health and well-being.

I have come across a "liberation pledge" that you can take as a form of activism or an impactful way of standing up for your beliefs. This pledge consists of publicly living vegan, publicly refusing to eat where animals are being eaten, and openly encouraging others to take the pledge. [1]This pledge aims to create a new societal norm: animals are not here for humans to use. Taking the oath may help you, or it may not. It all depends entirely on who you are, what works for you, and your boundaries. Refusing to be around those who are eating animals can undoubtedly be isolating at first, so it may only be something you choose to take on down the road, or not at all.

Can I still call myself vegan if I have to take non-vegan medication?

To answer this question, I usually refer to the official definition of veganism as put forward by The Vegan Society:

> *"Veganism is a way of living which seeks to exclude, as far as is possible and practicable, all forms of exploitation of, and cruelty to, animals for food, clothing or any other purpose."*

Pay close attention to the statement *"as far as is possible and practicable"* – this footnote covers all forms of animal exploitation that are impossible (or near to impossible) to avoid in a non-vegan society. I would argue that medication does fall under this category. Nobody should neglect or forsake their health for the (mostly fictional) vegan "purity" concept. What is cruel, unnecessary, and avoidable should be avoided – the rest cannot yet be helped. So, if the medication you need is coated with lactose or gelatin, it's tested on animals, and there is no other option currently available, then you should be taking it free of guilt. We can only trust that, in the future, the world at large will become more vegan-friendly than it is now.

Can dogs and cats eat vegan as well?

This question is a controversial one. For cats, I'm sure you've come across some of those clickbait articles claiming that vegans are trying to get their cats to eat like them, leading to the exact opposite scenario that veganism preaches: animal cruelty. While any specific group of people will have some bad apples, I can safely say I've never met, or even spoken to, a vegan trying to feed a vegan diet to their cat. Cats cannot eat a plant-based diet under any circumstance, as just like their distant tiger and lion cousins, they are natural carnivores. Vegans who wish to own cats will have to come to terms with the fact that they will have to purchase animal products to feed their pets. If this is something that you, as a vegan, are not willing to compromise on, you should probably rethink your decision. Conversely, if you or your family already have a furry friend living in the household, that compromise must be made.

Dogs are omnivores, and they can be happy and healthy on a plant-based diet.[2] But you shouldn't just feed your dog your vegan leftovers – your furry companion's diet should be planned cautiously and consciously, making sure to consult a veterinary nutritionist before making any decisions. Vegan dog food brands like *V-dog* and *Wild Earth* are available online for you to purchase in bulk, and websites like *veggiepets.com* can give you an in-depth understanding of what your dog should eat to thrive, not just survive, on a plant-based diet. After all, the foods are specially formulated to meet your dog's nutrition requirements.

Is a vegan diet safe for toddlers and children?

From pregnancy to birth, breastfeeding, the first birthday, and beyond, a vegan diet is suitable for all life stages. Children can get everything they need for their development by following a vegan diet. The parents must be well informed and conscious of where nutritional inadequacies might stem from. Essential vitamins and minerals like vitamin D, omega-3 fatty acids, calcium, iron, and vitamin B_{12} are crucial for vegans of all ages and even more so for newborns, toddlers, and children.[3]

I was vegan throughout my second pregnancy, and my experience wasn't in any way different from what all women go through: morning sickness, cravings, food avoidance, an increased dosage of essential vitamins. My children are growing up eating the same way I do, though getting them to eat their vegetables can sometimes be a struggle (yes, even vegan children will fight tooth and nail so that they don't have to eat their broccoli and spinach). They love avocados, roasted chickpeas, bananas, peas, and pasta – they're just like any other children, and they are growing up just as healthy as their omnivore peers, if not much more. As a parent, I fully understand how worried some might be regarding their children's well-being. Still, the research is crystal clear: a vegan diet is suitable for people of all ages, as long as their nutritional needs are considered.

COMMON ARGUMENTS AND HOW TO RESPOND

*I*t's no secret – vegans face a lot of criticism.

And it's easy to figure out why. People will build a wall between you and them, creating arguments that are either understandable (stemming from confusion and lack of knowledge) or merely grasping at straws to mask their discomfort with the ethical questioning you are sparking in them by simply being yourself. Whether you are actively bringing up the topic or not, you are challenging how they've done things their whole life by just being a vegan, and most people don't want to hear that they are hurting others - even when they're not fully conscious of it.

That being said, I want to give some examples of arguments you may hear from those around you and some answers you can give them in return. One tip when replying to people's questions (if you choose to engage at all, it is your choice after all) is to be quick and to the point. Keep in mind that some people aren't looking for an answer to get a rise out of you. In other cases, they are operating from a place of curiosity and genuine interest in a lifestyle that seems too foreign and unattainable. Keep in mind that coming from a place of love and understanding will get you farther than putting up a wall and becoming defensive. Leading by example is one of the best ways to inspire others and show that a vegan lifestyle is viable and one you can thrive on.

Everyone is on a personal journey, and you have to keep in mind that not that long ago, you might not have been that different from the people confronting you now. I think it's quite valuable to remember that most of us come from the same diet and lifestyle, one that assumes animals are ours to use and exploit. A tiny bit of empathy will work wonders in helping us connect with people who don't understand veganism just yet.

You were once in their shoes too – perhaps, even a few chapters ago.

It's my personal choice to eat what I want!

If there is a victim involved, it's no longer a personal choice.

This is an age-old question, the debate on where your freedom ends and where another being's freedom begins. Animals have their choice of freedom taken away when forced into this endless cycle of human consumption, a tragic fate they cannot opt-out of from the day they are born. The vast majority of people are led to believe that their personal choice does not impact others. Still, we are raised to believe animal exploitation is an unavoidable part of life. We are so far removed from the slaughter process behind closed doors that we don't make the connection until we choose to. If you've heard the saying "*igno-rance is bliss*" before, well - this is precisely the sort of situation it would apply to. If you choose to ignore what's happening or choose to remain ignorant of the suffering that puts food on your plate, your heart cannot truly feel the pain of the living, breathing creatures we choose to take the life of.

So, in turn, yeah, I guess the choice of what we eat "only affects us" — but only because we routinely ignore that there is an "other" we are affecting through our self-serving choices.

Moreover, if exploiting animals for personal gain was indeed a legitimate choice, why choose to be cruel in the first place?

Where do you get your protein?

As discussed in length before this chapter, plants have all the essential amino acids you need to meet your daily protein requirements. It is not that much of a tall order when popular plant foods like beans, soy, and nuts are considered great protein sources by all dieticians.

A grown adult needs approximately 0.8 grams per kilogram of body weight, taking up 15% of our daily calorie requirements.[1] While this is supposed to be a minimum, note that excess protein is expelled from your body and not stored. The amount of protein our bodies need isn't as high as is commonly believed, and protein-packed plant foods have all you need for your body to thrive. The key is to incorporate the right amount of protein in all your meals or start the day with a fresh protein smoothie if you're having trouble planning balanced meals.

People commonly believe that protein comes only from animal products, especially meat products, which is understandable as that's what we've been told our whole life. But consider this: if all creatures need protein to live (which they do, though in varying amounts), then where are the plant-eating cows getting their protein from? What about bulls and the oxen we want to be as strong as? Their protein also comes from plants, of course.

Plants feel pain too!

This is scientifically untrue.

Plants have no central nervous system, and there is no scientific or empirical evidence showing that they suffer.[2] They will react to damage on a chemical level (for example, breaking down when you're mowing the lawn), but that doesn't mean they suffer.

I've never witnessed this argument being used seriously, but more of a surefire way of getting a rise out of vegans and vegetarians – don't fall for it.

Remain calm and present your conversational partner with the facts and a smile on your face. If they raise their concerns surrounding plants' wellbeing, have them consider the number of plants fed to animals raised for human consumption (it's a lot more than the plants any vegan eats daily). Ask them why they are still eating meat if they genuinely care about the suffering of plants. Spoiler alert – they will have nothing to say about it.

Vegans can't get enough (insert nutrient here).

As I mentioned before, the Academy of Nutrition and Dietetics (the largest body of diet and nutrition professionals in the U.S.) considers a vegan diet appropriately planned to be healthful, nutritionally adequate, and appropriate for every stage of life.

Some essential nutrients like iodine, vitamin B_{12}, omega-3 fatty acids, and vitamin D_3 might be harder to get by following a plant-based diet, but this doesn't mean that vegans won't have the means to get enough of these minerals. A proper multivitamin will take care of all your nutritional needs, whether you are vegan or not. In fact, I know some non-vegan nutritionists that deal with patients following all sorts of meat and animal product-heavy diets, and they come across vitamin deficiencies (B_{12} included) across the board. All diets carry a risk of nutrient deficiency if not appropriately planned, and vegan diets are certainly no exception to the rule. Eating whole foods regularly and incorporating daily supplements is crucial, whether you are a health-nut plant-based eater, a junk food vegan, or a person following a standard American diet packed with meat, eggs, and dairy products.

Humans have canines, so we are meant to eat meat.

This is a popular vegan-baiting argument that is nothing but a myth.

Compared to true carnivores like lions and bears, human canines are relatively flat, and they cannot rip through raw flesh as a lion's canines would. Not to mention the fact that primarily vegetarian animals like gorillas also display enormous canines – teeth you'd never see ripping through a prey's flesh. In the animal world, teeth are meant for breaking down food and a way to show dominance.[3] Showing teeth is a widely employed behavior in the animal kingdom to ward off threats; look at your family dog or cat.

Having canines does not necessarily equate to being a carnivore.

Further, take into account that human bodies are more closely related to herbivorous animals than carnivorous animals. We lack the claws and the sharp teeth, our intestines are longer than animal omnivores and carnivores,[4] our stomach acid is weaker than flesh-eating animals, and our jaws chew side to side rather than up and down. All these signs point to an herbivorous animal.

Finally, even if you are not ready to accept that nature did not "design us" as meat-eaters, consider this: what our bodies look like doesn't matter when trying to justify the way we treat animals. It doesn't mean we should do something just because we can — it doesn't make it okay.

Animals aren't sentient.

More blatant misinformation.

On one faithful day (*The Cambridge Declaration of Consciousness*), world-renowned neuroscientists and other great thinkers (one of whom was Stephen Hawking) concluded that animals are, in fact, sentient.[5] The textbook definition of sentient is "able to feel or perceive things," which we can all agree does apply to animals of all shapes and sizes.

I'm sure you have seen it yourself — animals do feel pain, love, and happiness. Just take your dog as an example. They will wag their tails when excited, growl when they're upset, and get scared of thunderstorms and fireworks.

Each animal has a language and way of responding to stimuli, but that doesn't mean they don't experience the world like us, though perhaps a little simpler, a little more visceral. Recognizing animal sentience is vital for us to know when animals are properly cared for, so they can live their fullest, happiest lives. Only when we realize this can we translate empathy into action, like rethinking the types of foods we eat.

I only eat humanely raised meat and cage-free eggs!

"Humane" meat and "humane" dairy and eggs are nothing but a marketing ploy.

The definition of humane is to show compassion or benevolence. I would attest that killing an animal (in any way and through any method) does the complete opposite of that. The harsh reality is that cage-free hens don't get to roam freely in a "happy" farm, calves don't get to drink their mother's milk, and slaughter is still slaughter, no matter the conditions farm animals were raised in before their lives are put to an end.

Is it morally justifiable to slaughter something that does not want to die?

Is it compassionate to kill another healthy, living being for no real reason but our gluttony, convenience, or tradition?

We can all understand that animals want to live and always choose life over death, freedom over entrapment, and pleasure over pain. So, when the idea of killing an animal "humanely" comes up, it's hard to understand how any method could achieve this. The humane way to do anything to an animal is to help it when it's hurt, free it when it's caged, and leave it alone to live its life.

If you were stranded on a deserted island, and the only thing to eat was a pig, would you eat it?

It might feel silly to defend a scenario that would never happen, but this is sadly one of the most prevalent challenges voiced by meat-eaters.

The situation presented here is one of survival, far removed from our day-to-day reality where we get to make our own choices free of survivalist pressure. No one knows how we will react in such extreme situations, but I would say that severe cases may call for actions we would not usually justify in regular society. So, how does this tragic scenario relate to our daily lives and behavior in everyday society as a whole? Well, it doesn't.

However, if we were to engage with this absurd scenario, how likely would it be that there'd be a lone pig on an entire island, healthy and living, without any plant food for it to eat? You could argue that you'd follow the pig around and look for the food it's eating and see how you could feed yourself in the same way to survive. The pig ultimately would just become a friend.

Finally, if you feel incredibly bold, you could even ask a straight-forward question: "If you were stranded on a deserted island, and the only thing to eat there was another person, would you eat them?".

LEAVE A REVIEW

If you enjoyed this book and found it helpful, consider leaving a review.

As a small independent company, we would really appreciate your feedback.

Thank you for being a reader of The Vegan Nook!

CONCLUSION

First of all, I'm so glad you have come to discover veganism. Whatever your background, whatever the reason behind your interest in adopting a plant-based diet and vegan lifestyle, you are making a decision that will impact the course of your entire life – and doing something like this takes guts.

It takes courage and humility to reflect upon your everyday actions and lifelong beliefs, deconstruct them, and transform how you see the world to make it a better place for your fellow humans and the animals. This truly is the beginning of the rest of your life, a new you, free of harmful traditions that do nothing but weigh us down, making us comfortable living the unexamined life. And yes, this is just the beginning: the shape and direction that your vegan journey takes is ultimately up to you. It might take you months or even years to get to the point where you feel comfortable calling yourself a vegan. You might decide to leave your old diet in the past, but continue purchasing other animal products in your lifestyle until you know the time is right to go further in your convictions. You might encounter unexpected challenges along the way, like a sudden move to a new place far removed from your vegan-friendly reality, a partner claiming they'll never go vegan (*never in a million years*), or an unexpected intolerance to soy and wheat products. The key is to keep moving forward – at your own pace, with pit stops and U-turns along the way, but always unmistakably forward.

Take the time you need to fully own your actions by revisiting your *why power* at different stages of your vegan journey. Carry out more research if you find you haven't fully grasped a key concept related to a cruelty-free life or happen to come across a brand-new idea that completely revolutionizes the principles you held to before. Remember that veganism is not a fixed philosophy or static dogma: many aspects of the lifestyle might become more open to interpretation or debate over time. The scientific community is continuously evolving to incorporate fresh discoveries into nutritional, environmental, and behavioral science. Once you have successfully learned all the basics from my suggested reading list and watchlist, do your best to keep up with your favorite vegan content creators and vegan-friendly media outlets to be in the know. Whether it's the latest animal welfare policy, the most recent environmental summit, or even just the newest dairy substitute to hit the plant-based market, do your part to stay informed and engaged in the community as time goes on. You might lose some friends over your choices, and that's okay – it says more about them than it does about you. The world is full of extraordinary, supportive individuals that will keep you growing into the best version of yourself you can be. Creating a strong community of like-minded vegans (or just ethically conscious people) will improve your life in a variety of ways you never thought were possible while making the world a better place at the same time.

If there was just one thing I wanted you to take away from this simple guide, it's that going vegan can be an immensely exciting journey. We often focus on the negative, on the challenges we will face trying to get closer to our ideals, on the things we will miss, and miss out on how we may fail. I am somewhat guilty of that, too, as, throughout this book, I have done my best to address concerns and fears that may arise as you become the vegan you want to be. After all, focusing on the negative and overthinking where our choices may lead us is a necessary part of the human condition. My main objective while writing down what I have learned has been to assuage those fears and doubts by giving you the tools and resources to make informed decisions.

But trust me, this is going to be fun. You will try so many new foods, connect with so many different people, travel to places you've never thought you would, and become a version of yourself you never thought was possible to achieve.

Veganism is growing like never before.

In the past eight years as a vegan, I have seen my local Starbucks go from being the last place I'd ever want to visit to offering an array of plant milk and vegan meals available for me during a day out.

Some of the challenges you might experience in your first few months as a vegan might no longer be there even just a year from now, and as I have made sure to cover most of those challenges throughout this book, I'm fairly sure you're in for a pretty smooth ride. Keep asking questions, keep doubting what you take for granted, and let your heart guide you by tuning into your empathy and compassion. Who knows, going vegan might open your mind to even more conscious decisions you can take as part of your journey: being aware of your overall carbon footprint, rethinking fast fashion, ditching plastic, repurposing and revamping rather than throwing it away.

But these are all just ideas, of course. When it comes to my personal experience, I realized that veganism opened the floodgates to a brand-new world of conscious choices I never considered before. It opened my eyes to a more purposeful way of living, one that I pledged would extend to more than just the food I put on my plate. My daily mantra is quite simple:

"Whatever it takes, just do what's right."

It's incredible how such a simple concept can impact the world so much, just by being *simply vegan.*

But at the end of the day, isn't that what being a vegan is all about?

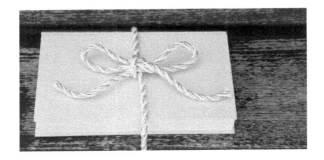

As a way to say thank you, we've put together The Essential Vegan Bundle, just for you.

Included are customizable recipes, the best resources and a grocer cheat sheet!

Click here for your bundle!

NOTES

1. ALLOW ME TO INTRODUCE YOU

1. Lactose intolerance - Genetics Home Reference - NIH. (2020, May 26). Retrieved June 1, 2020, from https://ghr.nlm.nih.gov/condition/lactose-intolerance

2. Butler, S. (2014, April 04). Beans and Greens: The History of Vegetarianism. Retrieved June 01, 2020, from https://www.history.com/news/beans-and-greens-the-history-of-vegetarianism

3. Is Sugar Vegan? (2018, August 08). Retrieved June 01, 2020, from https://www.peta.org/living/food/is-sugar-vegan/

4. Zampa, M. (2020, April 19). How Many Animals Are Killed for Food Every Day? Retrieved June 01, 2020, from https://sentientmedia.org/how-many-animals-are-killed-for-food-every-day/

5. New Study: Vegan Diet Reduces Carbon Footprint by 73% - Vegconomist, The vegan business magazine. (2019, July 19). Retrieved June 01, 2020, from https://vegconomist.com/society/new-study-vegan-diet-reduces-carbon-footprint-by-73/

6. United Nations. (2018, September 26). Tackling the world's most urgent problem: Meat. Retrieved June 01, 2020, from https://www.unenvironment.org/news-and-stories/story/tackling-worlds-most-urgent-problem-meat

7. Wasting water. (2012, March 26). Retrieved June 01, 2020, from https://www.ciwf.org.uk/research/environment/wasting-water/

8. Cameron, J., & Cameron, S. A. (2017, December 04). Animal agriculture is choking the Earth and making us sick. We must act now. The Guardian. Retrieved June 1, 2020, from https://www.theguardian.com/commentisfree/2017/dec/04/animal-agriculture-choking-earth-making-sick-climate-food-environmental-impact-james-cameron-suzy-amis-cameron

9. Margulis, S. (2004). Causes of Deforestation of the Brazilian Amazon. World Bank Working Paper No. 22. Washington, DC: World Bank. https://openknowledge.worldbank.org/handle/10986/15060

10. Cronin, A. M. (2016, June 01). You Can Save Over 200,000 Gallons of Water A Year with One Simple Choice. Retrieved June 01, 2020, from https://www.onegreenplanet.org/environment/how-to-save-water-with-one-simple-choice/

11. Veganism Impact Report. Retrieved June 01, 2020, from https://www.veganismimpactreport.com/

12. Poore, J., & Nemecek, T. (2018). Reducing food's environmental impacts through producers and consumers. Science, 360(6392), 987-992. doi:10.1126/science.aaq0216

13. Doyle, A. (2015, September 16). Ocean Fish Numbers Cut in Half Since 1970. Retrieved June 01, 2020, from https://www.scientificamerican.com/article/ocean-fish-numbers-cut-in-half-since-1970/

14. Kassam, S., Dr. (2019, June 20). Can a plant-based diet prevent or even reverse chronic disease? Retrieved June 01, 2020, from https://www.globalcause.co.uk/plant-based-alternatives/can-a-plant-based-diet-prevent-or-even-reverse-chronic-disease/#

15. Tonstad, S., Butler, T., Yan, R., & Fraser, G. E. (2009). Type of Vegetarian Diet, Body Weight, and Prevalence of Type 2 Diabetes. Diabetes Care, 32(5), 791-796. doi:10.2337/dc08-1886

16. Rizzo, N. (2013). Nutrient Profiles of Vegetarian and Nonvegetarian Dietary Patterns. Journal of the Academy of Nutrition and Dietetics, 113(12), 1610–1619. doi:10.1016/j.jand.2013.06.349

17. Plant-Based Diet Reverses Heart Disease. (2014, July 01). Retrieved June 01, 2020, from https://www.pcrm.org/news/health-nutrition/plant-based-diet-reverses-heart-disease

18. Melina V, Craig W, Levin S. Position of the Academy of Nutrition and Dietetics: Vegetarian Diets. Journal of the Academy of Nutrition and Dietetics (2016). 116(12):1970-1980. doi:10.1016/j.jand.2016.09.025

2. BE COMPASSIONATE TO YOU

1. Herzog, H. (2014, December 2). Retrieved from https://www.psychologytoday.com/intl/blog/animals-and-us/201412/84-vegetarians-and-vegans-return-meat-why

2. McLeod, S. A. (2018, June 06). Jean piaget's theory of cognitive development. Simply Psychology. https://www.simplypsychology.org/piaget.html

3. Cherry, K. (2020, February 19). Retrieved from https://www.verywellmind.com/what-is-a-confirmation bias-2795024#:~:text=A%20confirmation%20bias%20is%20a,creative%20than%20right%2Dhanded%20people

4. Walesh, S. (n.d.). Using the Power of Habits to Work Smarter. Retrieved June 10, 2020, from http://www.helpingyouengineeryourfuture.com/habits-work-smarter.htm

5. Herzog, H. (2014, December 2). Retrieved June 10, 2020, from https://www.psychologytoday.com/intl/blog/animals-and-us/201412/84-vegetarians-and-vegans-return-meat-why

6. Badiei, S. (2017, May 4). Retrieved from https://www.pickuplimes.com/single-post/2017/05/04/PANTRY-ESSENTIALS-»-printable-grocery-shopping-list

7. Hoppe, D. (2014, February 26). Retrieved June 10, 2020, from https://drdianahoppe.com/whats-your-why-power/

3. SETTING UP FOR SUCCESS

1. Duhigg, C. (2014). The power of habit: why we do what we do in life and business. New York: Random House Trade Paperbacks.

2. Lally, P., et al. (2010). How are habits formed: Modelling habit formation in the real world. European Journal of Social Psychology, 40, 998–1009. doi: 10.1002/ejsp.674

4. FOOD — THE GOOD STUFF

1. Tips for healthy eating. (2019, December 23). Retrieved June 10, 2020, from https://food-guide.canada.ca/en/tips-for-healthy-eating/make-healthy-meals-with-the-eat-well-plate/

2. Pendick, D. "How Much Protein Do You Need Every Day?" (2015, June 18). Retrieved June 10, 2020, from www.health.harvard.edu/blog/how-much-protein-do-you-need-every-day-201506188096

3. Medawar, E., Huhn, S., Villringer, A., & Veronica Witte, A. (2019). The effects of plant-based diets on the body and the brain: a systematic review. Translational psychiatry, 9(1), 226. doi:10.1038/s41398-019-0552-0

4. Felman, A. "Everything you need to know about vitamin B-12" (2017, November 28). Retrieved June 10, 2020, from https://www.medicalnewstoday.com/articles/219822

5. Thomas, D. (2003). A study on the mineral depletion of the foods available to us as a nation over the period 1940 to 1991. Nutr Health, 17(2), 85-115. doi:10.1177/026010600301700201

6. Gunnars, K. (2018, June 11). "How to Optimize Your Omega-6 to Omega-3 Ratio". Retrieved June 11, 2020, from https://www.healthline.com/nutrition/optimize-omega-6-omega-3-ratio

6. WHAT TO WATCH OUT FOR

1. Soteriou, H. (2018). Why you may have been eating insects your whole life. BBC News. Retrieved June 12, 2020, from https://www.bbc.co.uk/news/business-43786055#:~:text=This%20is%20be-cause%20one%20of,where%20they%20live%20on%20cacti.

2. Are animal ingredients included in white sugar? (2015, October 14). Retrieved June 18, 2020, from https://www.peta.org/about-peta/faq/are-animal-ingredients-included-in-white-sugar/

9. ANSWERING QUESTIONS YOU MAY HAVE

1. The Liberation Pledge. Retrieved June 27, 2020, from http://www.liberationpledge.com/

2. Heinze, C. (2016, July 21). Vegan Dogs - A healthy lifestyle or going against nature? Retrieved June 27, 2020, from https://vetnutrition.tufts.edu/2016/07/vegan-dogs-a-healthy-lifestyle-or-going-against-nature/

3. Vegetarian and vegan babies and children. (2019, February 27). Retrieved June 27, 2020, from https://www.nhs.uk/conditions/pregnancy-and-baby/vegetarian-vegan-children/

10. COMMON ARGUMENTS AND HOW TO RESPOND

1. Gunnars, K. (2018, July 05). Protein Intake - How Much Protein Should You Eat Per Day? Retrieved June 27, 2020, from https://www.healthline.com/nutrition/how-much-protein-per-day

2. Loria, J. (2018, June 15). Here's Why You're Wrong When You Say Plants Feel Pain. Retrieved June 27, 2020, from https://mercyforanimals.org/heres-why-youre--when-you-say-plants#:~:text=Plants%20have%20no%20brain%20or,they%20-can't%20feel%20anything.&text=Even%20though%20plants%20-don't,plant%20to%20start%20protecting%20itself

3. Lee, N., & Polan, S. (2019, March 08). Why humans have canine teeth. Retrieved June 27, 2020, from https://www.businessinsider.com/canine-teeth-sharp-front-apes-evolution-ancestors-2019-5?r=US&IR=T

4. Is It Really Natural? The Truth About Humans and Eating Meat (2018, January 23). Retrieved June 27, 2020, from https://www.peta.org/living/food/really-natural-truth-humans-eating-meat/#:~:text=Intesti-nal%20Length&text=Humans'%20intestinal%20tracts%20are%20-much,for%20humans%20to%20eat%20meat

5. Low, P. (2012, July 07). The Cambridge Declaration On Consciousness. Retrieved June 27, 2020, from http://fcmconference.org/img/CambridgeDeclarationOnConsciousness.pdf

Lightning Source UK Ltd.
Milton Keynes UK
UKHW010633040321
379777UK00001B/247